5 "S"s OF YOGA

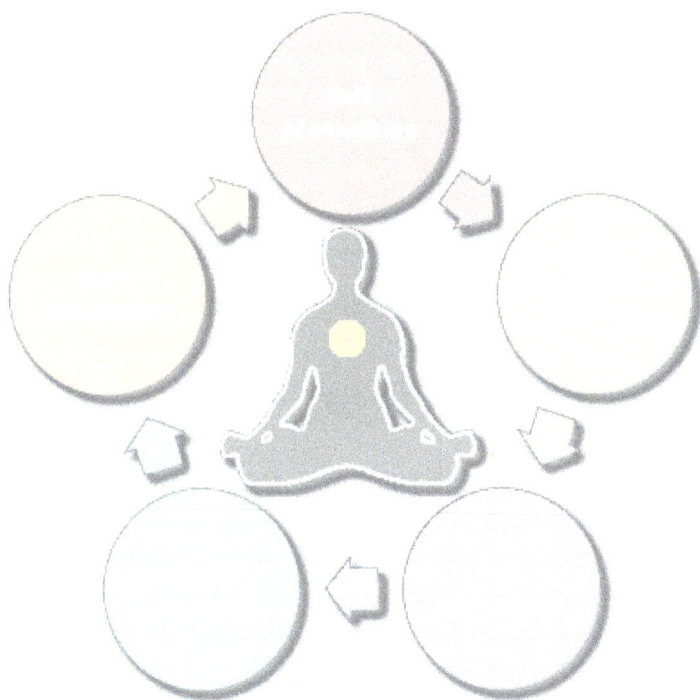

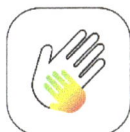

Newbee Publication

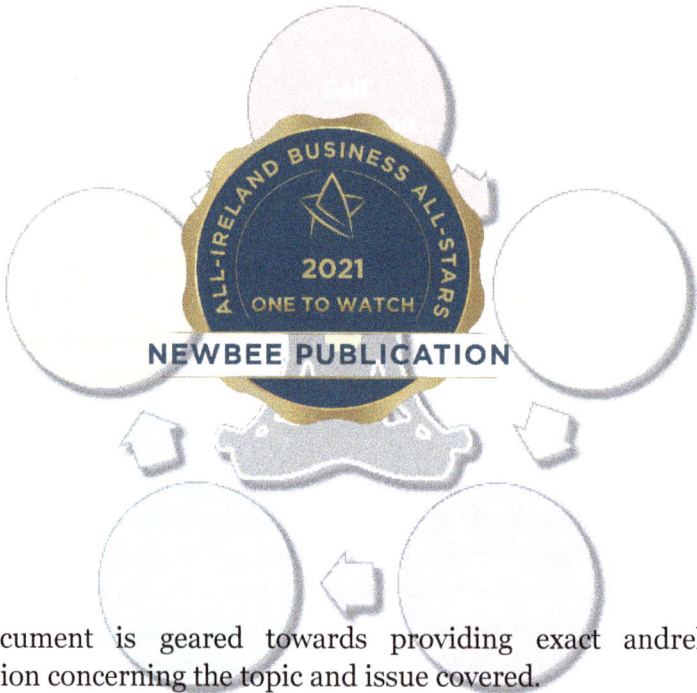

This document is geared towards providing exact andreliable information concerning the topic and issue covered.

It is not legal to reproduce, duplicate, or transmit any partof this document electronically or in printed format.

TABLE OF CONTENTS

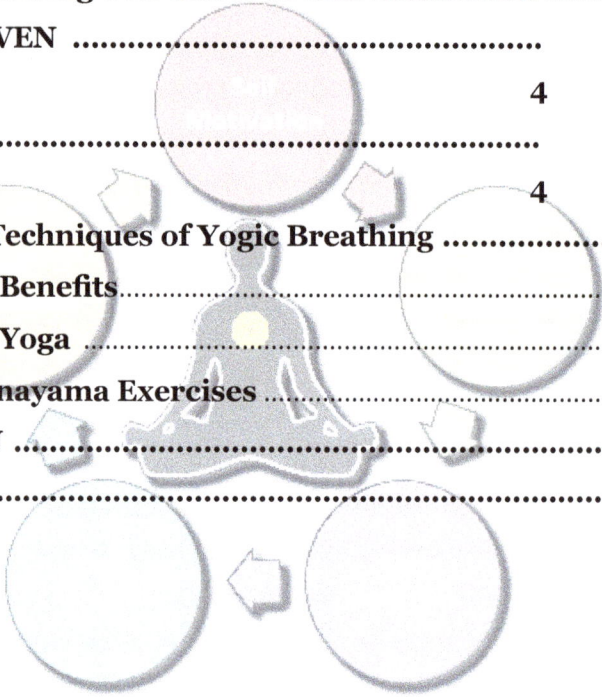

INTRODUCTION

Have you ever noticed that our creator made a super strong and super powerful machine - our body that can work non-stop for more than 100 years?

We can compare our bodies with the most modern, mobile, air-conditioned factory. Its building has a solid concrete structure built on pillars- the legs that give it movement. It has a nutrition production plant, air purification plant, circulation plant, filtration plant, reproduction plant, sewage plant, and top the head; It has an atomic reactor, super-computer, and telephone exchange, the fastest communication system compared to modern Apps and channels. It generates its own electricity and channelizes it according to the requirement of the factory. Surprisingly, all plants work automatically and incoordination.

This factory is built as a self-charging unit that means every single person's body on this earth can regulate itSELF. However, when we contravene natural rules by junk food, thoughts, and steps, we do not give the body a chance to regulate. Instead, we create toxins that the body attempts to get rid of in diseases and distress.

Yoga is a practice or strategy undertaken to fix and regulates the bodies corrupted systems and make us feel at peace within ourselves, free us from worries and anxieties. It eliminates or reduces the adverse effects of stress on the body, improving body awareness and overall well-being. According to Yogis, various benefits come with engaging in yoga, from physical to spiritual, mental, biochemical, and many more.

Yoga is defined as "the self-regulation of breath, focus on the body, and mind to achieve "unity in diversity," consciousness, and stillness of the body, tranquillity of the mind.

It is also known as the combination of the body and mind in union with the spirit.

Yoga has many beneficial physical properties that help the body to be more robust and more flexible. It also connects with the overall well-being of one's body, spiritual growth, and the ability to grow intellectually and rationally.

As a yoga teacher and practitioner, I explored different Yogic exercises associated with stretching and unwinding the muscles and attaining the body's poses (postures). After studying and practising yoga, I personally like Pranayama Yoga. Thus I have been running Pranayama yoga classes for the last 10 years. Pranayam Yoga is the mother of all kinds of yoga.

The most ancient form of yoga is performed by saints and great yogis.

Pranayama yoga is a breathing exercise that flows prana in the body.

Prana has several meanings: **breath, respiration, life, vitality, wind, energy, and strength**, while **Yama is restraint or discipline**. The control of prana leads to the mind's power, which is vital for concentration and meditation. But yogic breathing is also recognized to refresh and rejuvenate all the body systems. Breathing has excellent importance since yogic asanas or postures are mainly performed as per breathing.

As it is explained in Ayurveda that: "when breath wanders, the mind is unsteady, but when the breath is still, so as the mind still."

We can survive without food and water for a few days, but we cannot survive without breathing for more than five minutes. An individual breathes between 12-20 times per minute. If we take an average of 16 breaths per minute, that means we breathe about 960 breaths an hour, 23,040 breaths a day, 8,409,600 a year. Have you noticed that before, and how powerful is that?

Breathing is vital; we all knew about it, just the difference is that we are not aware of it. When we are doing pranayama yoga, we focus on breathing techniques. We think less about our worries and daily chores. This Process improves standard relaxation.

We can burn our mental experience as fuel when we exercise and reduce our body weight by consuming calories from our body fat.

Focusing on breathing practice while carrying out various poses (such as Siddhasana, Padmasana, or Shavasana) eliminates worries and stress. As a part of yoga, a key aspect is that it helps one be more focused and more concentrated. It also makes them more aware of their surroundings, making them more aware of the challenges they face.

As a part of the yoga practice, meditation techniques, such as mindfulness, can help us be more conscious of the body and feelings to a great extent and a great degree of the world around us. This brings about a great oneness and interdependency that helps unite the mind, body, and spirit. When meditation and breathing techniques are applied, we can achieve a calm and peaceful state within our minds and bodies in the way of Pranayama Yoga.

It is believed that there are several possible benefits of pranayama yoga; some of them are enumerated below:

1. Improves energy level

2. Boosts immunity

3. Enhances physical strength

4. Improves digestion and concentration power

5. Reduces fat around the abdomen

6. Makes the spine and waist more flexible.

7. Strengthens the muscles of arms, legs, and waist.

8. Make the heart and lungs stronger.

9. A secret of beautiful skin.

10. Improves blood circulation in the body.

11. It makes our body and brain function better.

12. Control blood pressure levels.

13. It tells the body to make the right hormones.

14. It gives more control over thoughts.

15. Stress levels stay down or low.

16. Help get rid of depression.

17. Help get rid of anger.

18. Helps in forgiving others and thinking big.

19. Helps to get rid of headaches & migraine.

20. Improve sleep pattern, helps to get rid of insomnia (try to do before going to bed or at the bed)

21. It creates space in your brain for new learning.

22. It improves memory span

23. It improves attention span and increaseslearning competence.

24. It changes mood and increases positivity.

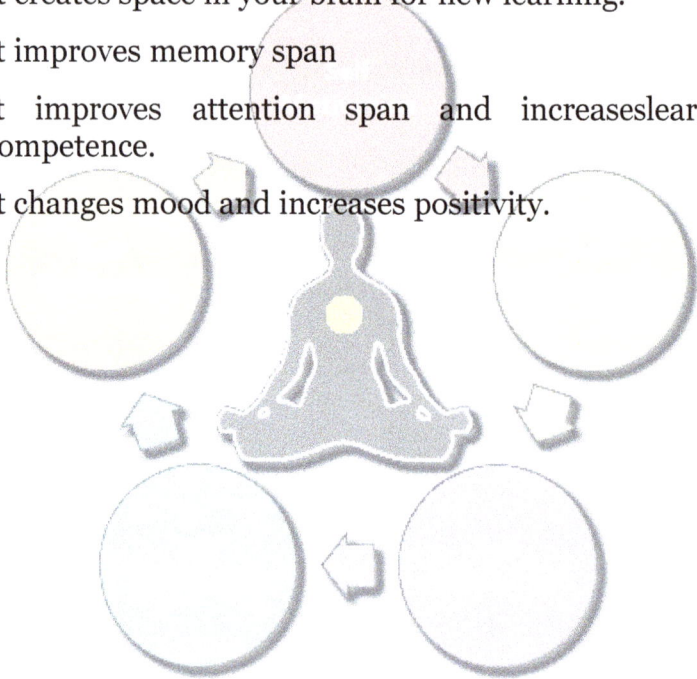

CHAPTER ONE

Understanding Yoga

Yoga is a discipline of the body and spirit that includes many postures (asanas). Yoga comes from the Sanskrit word jug, which means union of the individual consciousness with the universal consciousness. It is a personal development method and science of Indian spiritual practice born about 5000 years ago.

Yoga is good, but even if many people think yoga is just a set of physical exercises of twisting and stretching.

What distinguishes this discipline from gymnastics is searching for the body's harmony and spirit through stretching and strengthening postures (asana) and breathing techniques (Pranayama). This profound science that allows human to explore the human being's infinite potential soul.

The art of living yoga is a holistic lifestyle that integrates all the ancient knowledge of yoga: a discipline that unites the body, mind, and soul.

What is Yoga?

Yoga is an ancient Eastern practice that includes a wide variety of exercises and techniques.

The techniques used are:

- Physical postures, called Asanas.
- Respiratory practices: Pranayama.
- Deep meditation: Dharana and Dhyana.
- Deep relaxation: Yoga Nidra (sleep yoga).

Approach to Yoga

Since the late 19th century, it has been introduced to the West and has transformed a lot. There are 5 different modern yoga approaches, even if each type aims at global harmony by associating physical exercises with relaxation and meditation practices.

Here are the 5 approaches to modern yoga:

- Method of preventing disease and maintaining health - It is the most common form in the West. It is a revision of traditional Hatha Yoga and deals with the physical body (elasticity, endurance, and strength). The moral and spiritual aspects are not considered.
- As a sport, this yoga approach primarily exists in Latin America, although it is a very controversial concept. Yogis master hundreds of complex postures and even do contests.
- Body therapy. The practice of techniques to preserve health, body, and mind. This yoga practice is intended for therapeutic purposes.
- Complete lifestyle. Living this discipline means practising it daily (physical exercises or meditation) and applying yoga's wisdom daily.
- Spiritual discipline. You not only experience it as an integral part of your life, but you seek a spiritual dimension through meditative exercises.

Yoga: History

Yoga originated in India somewhere around 5000 BC in various forms & spiritual practices. Since then, it was passed from master to disciple over several generations. It is considered a science for the realization of the human being.

It was embraced by western culture approximately 100 years ago. Since then, it boomed around the late 1950s through numerous magazines and newspapers outlining its benefits to the general population.

Philosophy

2000 years ago, Patanjali wrote the first yoga text, Yoga Sutra, on practices and philosophy. He divided this discipline into 8 progressive stages that purify the body and mind and lead to enlightenment (samadhi). These stages are called the 8 arms; they must be understood and integrated into everyday life.

The 8 stages of yoga

Yama: Restraints, moral disciplines, or moral vows. It Includes moderation (non-violence on yourself or others, truth, honesty, and moderation in sexual life).

Niyama: Positive duties or observances, austerity, satisfaction, introspection of the body and soul.

Asana: the diversity of postures, kept motionless, activates breathing and concentration of the mind. The practice of Asanas helps to create and regenerate life energy.

Pranayama or breath control: Yoga is a physical, mental, and spiritual discipline. Pranayama Yoga and asanas go hand in hand. The union of these two Yogis principles is considered the highest form of purification and self-discipline covering both body and mind.

Practising inhalation and exhalation in a controlled manner will develop a relationship with the body, mind, and soul to align them in the centre.

Learning to breathe deeply and softly can:

- Calm the nervous system.
- Increase the volume of oxygen.
- Relax your muscles.
- Reduce tension and stress.

Pratyahara or control of the senses: by practising regularly, you can return to the essential by getting rid of the superfluous. So, you reach a state of deep consciousness. You can better live the present without thinking about the past or projecting yourself into the future.

Dharana or concentration: it is a practice that improves deep concentration.

Dhyana or meditation: meditation is the art of not doing and forgetting. Regular meditation practice helps you reconnect with your deep "self" and look at the world with peace of mind.

Samadhi: self-realization and enlightenment. Samadhi is t h e ultimate stage of yoga: overcoming your consciousness. You can achieve it when you lose the feeling of being a separate existence. Very few people reach this state, which Patanjali describes as the attainment of indescribable joy.

Health Benefits of Yoga

Yoga is a practice that seeks to work the body and mind in an interconnected way. It helps control stress, anxiety, pain, mood swings, and improve balance and promote a sense of overall well-being.

The most significant is that anyone can perform yoga; there is no age or strength limit. In my teaching, I use pranayama Yoga with gentle exercise and meditation. This combination suits all ages. There are young ladies in my group and ladies in their 80s, and they all love my yoga. They have experienced changes in their approach and behaviour towards life and everybody else in their lives.

It takes at least 3 months of practice to have all the benefits of yoga. As the person practices the activity, they can have greater body awareness and control the mind to influence the body. Thus, the whole organism operates in a harmonious and balanced manner.

1. Decreases stress and anxiety

The mind and the body are centred by yoga, which helps individuals concentrate on present situations. This gives the person a sense of peace and well-being in everyday life and dealing with problems that can arise daily.

This can ease depression by producing positive feelings, faster concentration, lowered irritability, and improved interpersonal relationships.

2. Promotes fitness

The exercises, techniques, and postures of this activity (being a Yoga instructor) can improve the muscles' resistance and strengthen.

Yoga helps to improve the body's performance for physical activities and daily tasks. It increases lean mass and leaves the body in shape, with more excellent definition and toned muscles.

3. Facilitates weight loss

One reason yoga can help you lose or maintain your weight is to control anxiety and binge eating.

Regular yoga can help to lose weight, but this is dependent on the style of practice.

Yoga practices burn fewer calories than traditional exercise (e.g., jogging, brisk walking). However, yoga can strengthen the body and increase mindfulness and how one relates to their body. So, individuals will become more aware.

4. Relieves bodily pain

Yoga can help you feel your body, which is called body awareness. With your increased body awareness, you will be more aware of your posture, how you walk, the way you sit, and the appearance of muscle tension. Doing so makes it possible to correct the body's bones, muscles, and joints to restore any changes. As a result, the musculoskeletal system is relaxed without damage to the bones and joints of the body. To help ease lower back pain, perhaps try some yoga exercises.

The posture and stretching exercises also help release tension and give the muscles flexibility, relieving pain.

In one study, individuals with carpal tunnel syndrome either received a wrist splint or did yoga for eight weeks. In the end, they found out that yoga was more effective in reducing pain and improving grip strength than wrist splinting.

5. Betters your bone health

The weight-bearing exercise of yoga strengthens bones because many yoga postures require that you lift your own weight.

An unpublished study conducted at California State University, Los Angeles (Ref:wikibooks.org) mentioned that yoga practice increased bone density in the vertebrae. In addition, yoga lowers the stress hormone cortisol may help keep calcium in the bones.

6. Drains your lymph nodes and boosts immunity

Lymph glands help clear the toxins from the body by removing the dead cells from the system. When you contract, stretch, move around, you help in the drainage system.

7. *Controls pressure and heart rate*

In addition to balancing the endocrine system, yoga enhances heart and lung functioning. It regulates the nervous system, improves blood circulation, heartbeat, blood pressure, and controls stress hormones cortisol adrenaline levels.

With proper treatment, lung expansion and breathing control exercises can result in better lung capacity. Yoga produces a different way for an individual to improve aerobic capabilities, such as increasing muscular stamina, flexibility, or strength.

8. Improves respiratory functions (lungs Capacity) and blood flow:

Pranayam yoga improves respiratory functions and increases lung capacity; even short-term yoga practice enhances lung capacity. This is because deep breathing provides a chance for tiny air sacs of the lungs to expand fully.

Yoga improves your blood flow in the body. By different posture, Yoga also gets more oxygen to your cells, helping them function better.

An article is mentioned in the International Journal of Yoga. A study is done by a group of researchers.

The study aimed to assess the effects of 8 weeks of asana and asana with pranayama lessons to clarify the influence of two different combinations of yoga practice on respiratory functions. (Ref.-International Journal of Yoga)

A total of 28 participants were divided into a yoga *asana* group A and a Yoga asana with *pranayama* group P. Participants attended 70-min session once a week for 8 weeks. The A group practised basic *asana* without specific breathing instructions. In contrast, the P group practised basic *asana* with specific breathing instructions (*pranayama*).

Both groups showed significant improvements in physical and overall respiratory functions after the 8-week yoga intervention. However, the maximum improvement was found in the P group.

9. Improves sleep

Yoga has been shown to increase melatonin production. This hormone regulates the sleep cycle, leaving you with more quality and depth.

By living a more relaxed and restful life, your body can also reflect this, waking up with more energy and disposition.

10. Improves pleasure in intimate contact

Sexual performance can also improve by doing yoga, as the couple's ability to relax and have better receptivity to the partner improves.

Controlling the concentration and alleviating anxiety, premature ejaculation, difficulty reaching orgasm, and erectile dysfunction can be controlled.

Health Benefits for the Elderly

Older people can benefit greatly from this activity's practice. It strengthens the muscles, relieves pain throughout the body, and improves balance, flexibility, and attention. The control of pressure, heart rate, and breathing is also affected by yoga, bringing a better quality of life and well-being to the elderly.

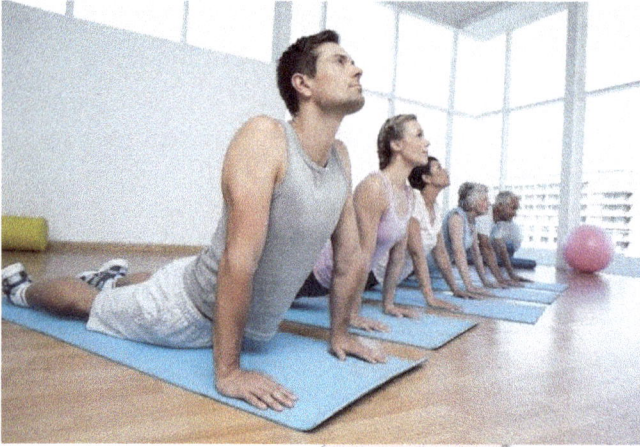

It is important to remember that the exercises practised in this activity must be adapted to each person's conditions and needs to do naturally and according to the benefits that the person seeks, thus avoiding injuries, sprains, or feelings of discouragement.

Benefits for Pregnant Women

In addition to being beneficial for any woman, yoga can also bring significant benefits during pregnancy. It improves flexibility and facilitates adaptation to changes in the body during this period, toning muscles, stretching joints, and making pregnancy less painful and tense. Besides, respiratory movements are also more synchronised, reducing shortness of breath in the final pregnancy periods.

The relaxation provided by being active can also reduce anxiety and worry, which are very common in pregnant women, making them calmer and facilitating the baby's development healthy. Physical exercises should be guided by a health professional during this period and released by the obstetrician, preferably light and relaxing.

It has also been noticed that the pregnant women who perform yoga before and after the delivery have fewer chances to get into Pre & postnatal depression.

Health Benefits in children:

There are many benefits of yoga if it introduces at the early stages of life. The primary believed advantages of yoga in children are.

- It increases Children's physical strength like - flexibility, balance, coordination, and muscle power.

- It improves children' focus, attention, concentration, memory span, learning power and retention of new information.

- It positively impacts children's social and psychological development by developing self-esteem, self-confidence, efficacy, and body awareness.

- It helps in self-reflection and whole-brain processing speed.

- It improves the capacities of the brain by recharging and restarting systems of body and mind.

- It creates new spaces in the brain by deleting old corrupted/painful/useless files.

- It creates a calm and relaxing environment that energises and nourishes, and integrates the central nervous system.

- It helps to dissipate tensions, reduce stress, and rebalance all systems of the body.

- It helps in reducing the feeling of helplessness, aggression, emotional and hormonal imbalance.

- It helps in improving academic performance as well as attitude towards themselves.

This book is a **self-help guide** to invest in ourselves and achieve desirable benefits.

When you are in the aeroplane, crew members instruct you about safety features and emergency procedures at the start. For example, they say that the panel above the head will open and reveal the oxygen masks in a change in cabin pressure.

The tag line is – "Remember to secure your own mask before assisting others."

The main reason for this is that you can only help your family and friends when you are healthy & safe yourself. If you run out of air, you cannot help anyone. Do not move forward to help others at the cost of your own life. But the irony is that we all are doing that in our daily lives. We are not giving attention to our health; we are all running around the clock without taking time to breathe. Finally, one day the body gives up and starts running out of air. That stage is when you begin to experience different mental problems, commonly known as anxiety, depression, insomnia, agitation etc. We need to attend ourselves first to be physically, emotionally, intellectually, and spiritually present to others.

This book is about achieving five "S" of yoga and its importance in our life.

The five "s" are

Self-discipline Self-

Control

Self- motivation Self- healing Self-realization

They all are interconnected. If you achieve one, the other one will gravitate towards you. The magnetic connections are made when you practice Pranayama yoga in your daily routine. Therefore, it is essential to understand what these S's are and why they are necessary for our life. Chapter seven describes- a set of Pranayama yoga exercises that you can incorporate in your daily life to achieve five S.

CHAPTER TWO
Self-Discipline and Yoga

Self-discipline is the first and second stage of yoga " Yama & Niyama", including the body's discipline, senses, and mind.

Through discipline, the body, the senses, and the mind are brought under control. Asanas, Pranayama, Pratyahara, Dharana, and dhyana are aids in the practice of self-discipline. Emotions and impulses are kept entirely under control.

To Achieve self-discipline, we need to kindle the inner fire. It is the union of the fire of the heart and the fire of the higher mind in a fiery aspiration towards the soul's light.

All discipline in yoga is self-discipline, which involves an effort to remember the aspiration and intention you are or decide to practice yoga. It does not include doing something because you have been told or because you must obey without understanding. Instead, you learn to use and apply them according to the circumstances with the tools and techniques you know to use from your knowledge.

In yoga, the fundamental thing is that what you are learning, experience for yourself, and use will improve the circumstances by reducing conditioning and habits.

It is not so much about how much I do but about the quality of what I do. Discipline should not create a rigid structure or tension or fall into feelings of guilt for not doing. Instead, it should be a feeling of pride in practising.

Discipline in yoga involves, above all, disciplining thoughts and attitudes so that they are reflected in actions. At first, the effort is to get out of mechanical conditioning habits and learn to think and know—rethinking relationships in another way, more creative and unrestrained.

The memory and the alignment with the essential spiritual intention and the group's energy strengthen the will, with yoga's activities and practices as priorities in life. Since that constant memory of the essence makes one renounce what is not essential and not feedback negative aspects, not beneficial relationships.

Discipline is the spiritual rhythm, and in this sense, it is not a duty; it is a right. Discipline, when enjoyed, is consecration. To consecrate is to make each act sacred since one is in contact with the inner being. In consecration, life is lived like a sacred ritual.

In the beginning, the effort should not focus on doing outside of every day, but on taking advantage of every day as possibilities of doing yoga. With the practice in groups, this effort makes a space of practice beyond obedient voluntarism incorporated into everyday life. This space creates a personal and intimate atmosphere where the practice takes on a unique feeling and meaning. It is where you learn to adapt yoga to your needs and not the other way around.

It is essential to develop a love relationship with yoga practice. When you love someone, you cannot live a single day without them; you feel anxious if they are not around. It feels like your life's energy is gone out of the body and nothing seem excellent or worthy. Like any relationship, if there is a doubt, get ready for the funeral of that relationship. You need to develop this relationship with yoga where you love being in Yoga without any doubts and tension.

The best way to see if we are progressing on the yoga path is through relationships. If our relationships improve in quality, clarity, and freedom, it is a good indication that our practice is well channelled; otherwise, we must review and ask ourselves what the cause, attitude, thought, or that relationship creates disharmony? And what technique or tool can I use to create a different result? Take advantage of conflicts to review intentions, attitudes, and thoughts that have generated them and try to change strategies to find them to create a more positive and harmonious relationship.

It is about living as apprentices and stop being victims. In victimhood, in the circle of guilt, we do not learn. We generate vicious circles where the same situations and conflicts are repeated in one way or another, without meaning.

Affirming the intention, remembering the sensations associated with it is the basis of discipline. That is the effort so that all practice has a heart. Understanding with a heart and the precise knowledge of the tools is the basis of all practice.

They are the ingredients that develop our aspirations and strengthen our search. One is harmonising with spiritual practice and their daily activity. Therefore, in their inner heart, they stop living them as something separate.

How to Practice Self-Discipline?

DEFINE YOUR GOAL: you might have heard it before to start by setting a small smart goal -specific, measurable, achievable, relevant, and time-bound.

To achieve that, sit at the same place simultaneously for the same duration for yoga and meditation. Starting with tangible things helps us to acquire the ability to be disciplined. That does not mean you do not have long-term goals; it helps to have a beacon at the end of the road, but it often happens that we end up giving up halfway by setting such ambitious goals. So, step by step, you do not want to run—one grain of sand at a time.

IDENTIFY DISTRACTORS: Today, there are many distractors around social networks, the Internet, television, advertising, etc. And the idea is not to rush out to buy a plane ticket to the Himalayas and abstract ourselves from the world. It is about learning to live in chaos and remain level-headed. Let us start by being honest with ourselves and identifying what things in our day are a distraction from what we have set out to do.

SPEND TIME: This point is the most important of all, from my perspective. Most of the time, we spend it complaining that we do not have enough time to do what we like, without realising that we could do more things that we enjoy by being more disciplined. It is a vicious cycle that we enter.

So, set a space in your schedule for the **next 21 days** (it is said that if you carry out a consecutive activity for 21 days, it becomes a habit) and decide the time you will dedicate to that first goal.

It is ideal for getting up early and making time for yoga and meditation. There are significantly fewer distractions in the morning, a quiet and peaceful environment, and fresh air. To stick with the smart goal, be disciplined, start with 10 minutes, and slowly increase the time.

BEGINS!!! It seems obvious, but do not believe it. How many times have you started planning to make a change in your life with great enthusiasm and the illusion only lasts a couple of hours, and you end up doing nothing? I am sure several times. Imagine your life as a video game, where you start with simple goals (which are the first worlds). As you progress and achieve those goals, the world's become more complicated and challenging. Take that first step, which will change the way you perceive the world.

REWARD YOURSELF: There will be those who agree with me and those who do not, but I think this is an integral part of learning to recognise our efforts and celebrate them. It does not have to be expensive or goes against what you are working on in the discipline, but it comforts you and values willpower and effort.

BE COMPASSIONATE: And yes, we must be realistic; there will be times when we will falter, where temptations, excuses and distractions can beat us in our race to have control of our lives in our hands. If that happens, nothing happens. Being compassionate with you means that: do not get angry, do not get frustrated, do not swear at yourself, do not get discouraged, do not quit. Remove all negative words from your dictionary and change with a positive affirmation like – I love to get up early for my 10 minutes yoga ritual. Remind yourself before going to bed, let your brain and body clock talk to in the night and assist you in the morning like a sentry.

Within yourself, you will find the strength to move forward. You will understand that falls and mistakes we can all have, but only those who desire to make things change are the ones who change their world.

DO NOT STOP: It means that once you have reached your first goal and it has made a habit of you, move on to the next one. As you progress, your discipline will manifest itself. You will be able to set yourself more complicated, more challenging tasks.

Discipline That Helps You Balance Body and Mind

Yoga is a very complete traditional discipline that seeks the connection between the body and the mind. Release stress by practising your asanas and meditating.

Stop. Breathe. Relax. Connect with yourself. Get rid of the stress of the day. A traditional discipline that seeks the union between the body and the mind in the present moment. An ideal practice for those who want to achieve a state of calm and concentration. Since its origins in India, Yoga has evolved and divided into various streams. There are many yoga disciplines widespread throughout the world, combining physical exertion and meditation.

Pranayama Yoga differs from the others because its practice includes:

- Prana (control of vital energy).
- Asanas (physical postures).
- Pratyahara (withdrawing from your sense).
- Dhyana (meditation).
- Samadhi (integration).
- Dharana (concentration).

All this makes Pranayama Yoga a very complete and harmonious discipline. It brings strength and lightness; combines expansion with submission; It fills us with energy but calms us down. Most yoga styles practised today, such as Vinyasa, Anusara, Hatha or Ashtanga, have their roots in Pranayama Yoga. It is the purest and most traditional discipline of all of them. Therefore, when starting to practice yoga, it is advisable to lay the foundations.

Anyone, regardless of age or physical condition, can practice it. Yoga is not demanding; everyone goes as far as they can.

Some of the asanas that promote self-discipline are the cobra, camel, angle, and triangle pose; in these asanas, our naval (solar plexus) is stretched and becomes the body's centre against gravity. The solar plexus is also known as "Nabhi Chakra", the controlling centre for all the organs below the diaphragm. This concept of Nabhi Chakra is not found in any other therapies except in "Ayurved", the Indian medicine of life. Shifting of solar plexus alignment leads to the disturbance in the organs below the diaphragm, so strengthening the solar plexus is most important.

Some asanas to create calmness in the body are the **tree's posture, the child, or the corpse**. Among the benefits of yoga, we may find:

- State of inner peace
- Enhanced heart and lung capacity
- Improved circulation
- Increased strength and endurance
- Increased flexibility
- Improved breathing
- Stress reduction

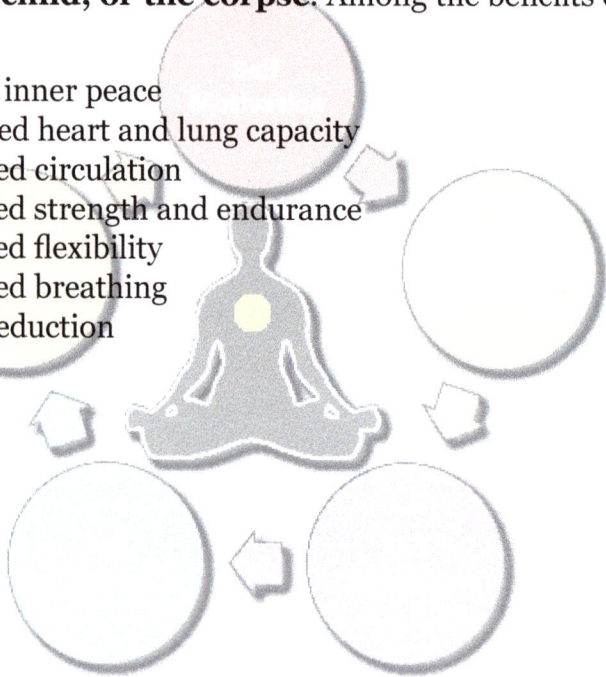

Triangles pose:

Stand straight and tall with your legs apart. Breath in & raise your arms at your side, slowly turn one side, and try to touch your foot. Bend as much as you can, do not force yourself; if you cannot reach to foot or ankle, just touch your shin. Turn your face towards the ceiling and look at the ceiling.

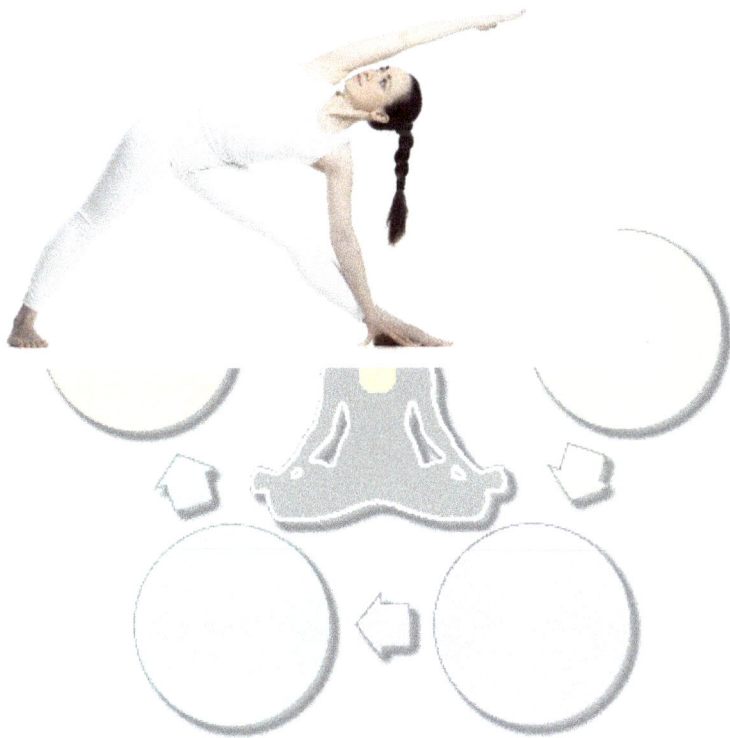

Child Pose:

Sit on your ankles (vajra asana) and breath-in, stretch your arms over your head, and breathe out while bending forward. Hold the position as long as you can, then slowly back to vajra asana.

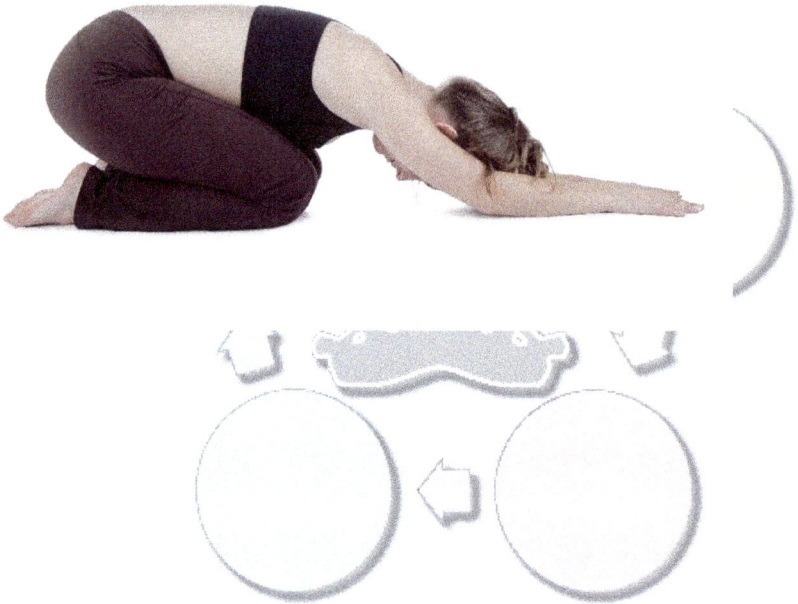

Camel pose:

Sit in vajra asana, hold your ankles with your arms and then slowly stretch your body. Look at the ceiling; maintain the posture if you can.

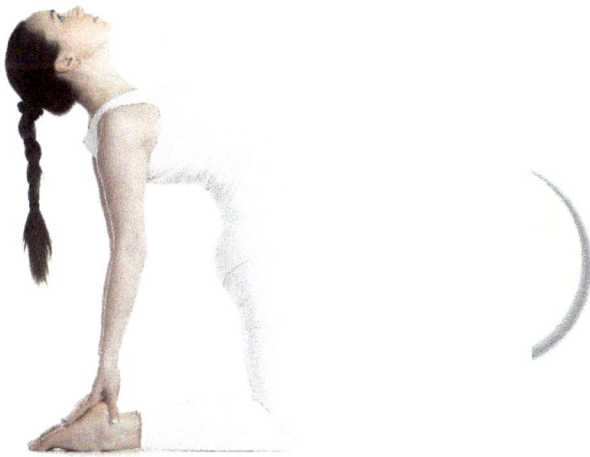

The ideal is to practice it once a day; however, each can start little by little and at their own pace. You can do it anywhere. Over time, the body   l
ask you   r
more,   d
you will
benefits.

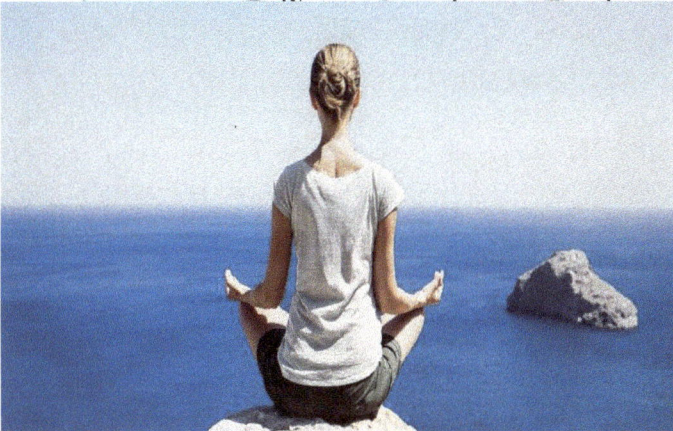

CHAPTER THREE
Self-Control and Yoga

Self-control is the fifth stage of yoga, "Pratyahara – control of the senses". Yoga ability to rein in our emotions and control our thoughts, actions, and desires. For example, you set a discipline to get up in the morning for your 10 minutes yoga ritual. You keep ongoing for a few days. One day, you start to procrastinate or come under the control of your desire to sleep more. Your lazy body produces a sound of solace, and you love to have it in that comfort zone. Your comforting thoughts create a signal to your mind, and your mind starts to react to your desire; it forces you to the action of skipping a day or two. You can achieve anything when you are 100 % committed or self-controlled.

We appeal to our capacity for self-control when, for example, we need to focus on a task without getting distracted. But we often do not make it? How can we strengthen self-control? What aspects should we keep in mind?

Our emotions help us respond adequately to stimuli according to our culture and what happens. However, when we experience it for long and let ourselves be carried away by it. It leads us to take actions that we then regret, undermining our self-esteem and becoming an obstacle to achieving our goals.

Therefore, it is essential to reflect on it, have the courage to question it, and face its answers.

Emotions like Anger comes when faced with a fact that makes us feel frustrated and prevents us from distinguishing Thoughts and actions. It usually relates to aggression suffered, whether real or not or limiting our desires and rights. Let us take sufficient time to analyse what we feel inside ourselves. We will notice that anger covers other emotions, such as sadness following a disappointment or even the fear of suffering.

We often tend to relate the word self-control only with the limitation of inconvenient behaviour. However, working on this skill also means taking on attitudes that positively influence the likelihood and the way things happen.

You need to understand the circle of your control

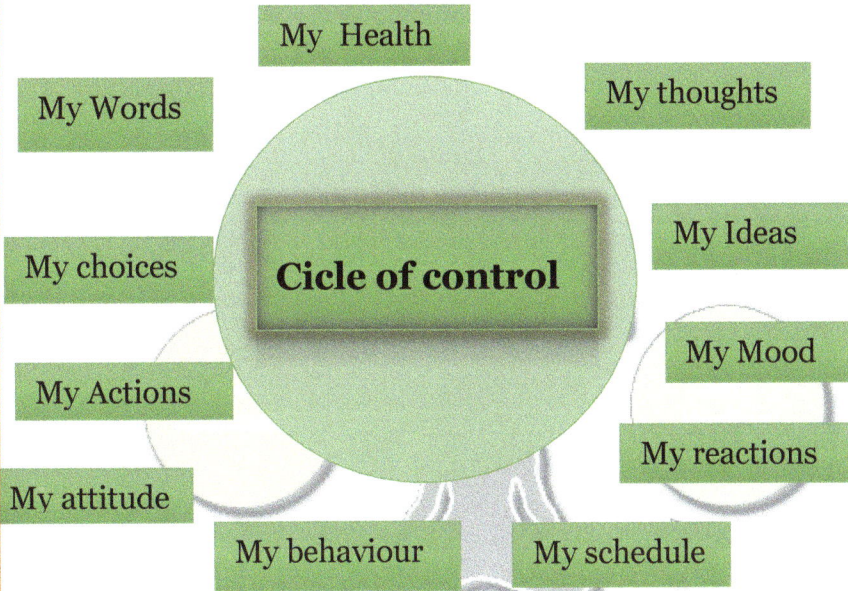

My Health

My thoughts

My Words

My Ideas

My choices

Cicle of control

My Mood

My Actions

My reactions

My attitude

My behaviour

My schedule

These things you can control. It is in your hands, but some things are not in your control.

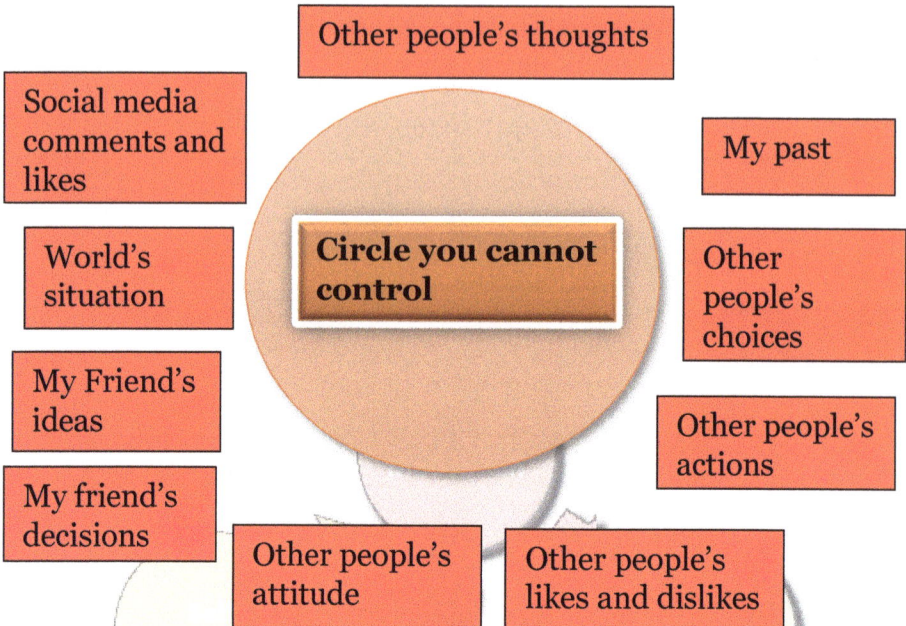

Other people's thoughts

Social media comments and likes

My past

Circle you cannot control

World's situation

Other people's choices

My Friend's ideas

Other people's actions

My friend's decisions

Other people's attitude

Other people's likes and dislikes

You can not control all these things, and there is a waste of your time and your brain's storage capacity for these things.

Your brain is like a hard drive. It can store unlimited data or files, but it will slow down your brain's processing time when your drive is filled with all uncontrollable junk files. As a result, you start forgetting things, and it changes your mood and increases irritability.

It is imperative to learn that emotions like anger clouded our thoughts, and we cannot think straight, so we cannot find the solution to the problem.

It is ideal not to go to bed angry; It will spoil your night as well as your following day. If you are angry and frustrated, the perfect thing is to get away from that situation into fresh air if possible and use the same code 6-2-7. It will change your brain's chemistry and refresh your brain.   Anger is an emotional reaction to unfulfilled desires and affairs. Anger is not a step to solve the problem. Anger is positive only when it is natural, negative when it arises from the imagination of one's mind tending to be destructive to oneself.

When you work on feelings, you will substantially change problematic situations by taking on a new attitude. Strengthening self-control is a path of understanding and connection with our way of conceiving the world, thoughts, feelings, and actions.

How Yoga Can Help Control extreme emotions:

It often happens that you need to control extreme emotions at the least opportune times or do not have the resources. When was the last time you felt angry? Do you remember the reason? Were you angry at yourself or someone else? Let us discover the source of anger and how yoga can help you manage it effectively.

To know the root of anger, we need to go back to the beginning. Have you seen a newborn baby show its anger? If you observe this phenomenon, you will notice that it does so in the least controlled way, throwing objects in the air and screaming. This shows that anger is an innate emotion that we often cannot control or manage, facing problems and conflicts with our loved ones or everyday life. Yoga and meditation can help you bring your awareness back to the centre and control your anger instincts.

"By cultivating [...] indifference towards miserable people, the mind keeps its calm undisturbed" (Sutra 1.33)

Patanjali, Yoga Sutra

Extreme emotions have primordial origins; they prepare the body and mind for a fight & flight. If you think about it without anger, you will not face the necessary determination and energy challenges, assert your rights, and maintain self-esteem.

Human beings are naturally led to exaggerate problems by always seeing them as more significant and insurmountable. Anger reveals itself dangerously and aggressively.

Study yourself in situations where you realise that anxious moods and anger predominate your well-being. Pay attention to the details of the situation and note what is happening by writing it detached. Rereading your experience of anger in the future will help you find solutions to new problems.

Believe in something bigger than you. Developing feelings of benevolence and tenderness towards the world and thinking of universal order contributes to maintaining a stable and peaceful state of mind by removing anger and pain.

Practice Yoga, asanas awaken the body and stimulate it to see the world from another perspective.

Yoga Poses to improve Self- Control

Nature has provided regulators and protectors in the body. These are the endocrine glands. Yogis in India were aware of it, working even before Ayurveda 6000 years ago and have described them in Chakras.

Sahastrar (Pineal- situated at the top centre of forehead)

Ajna (Pituitary – at the centre of the forehead between two eyebrows)

Vishudha (Thyroid/Parathyroid – located in the throat)

Anahat (Thymus glands – at heart)

Manipur (Adrenal and pancreas -Solar plexus - navel)

Swadhisthan (sex/gonads – 2 inches below the navel) Muladhara

(Root chakra- the base of the spine- tailbone area) These main endocrine glands produce internal secretion. Getting mixed with blood builds up the body, mind and maintains it in a healthy condition. These seven glands are interrelated and dependent on each other and assist each other. So all glands must work properly.

Yogis have shown that these endocrine glands-chakras also mould the mind and character. The Chakras play an essential role in developing the body and eliminating toxins from the body. But it also helps build human qualities like – affection, love, the capacity of higher thinking and concentration, leading to s e l f - c o n t r o l - balanced temperament, purity of heart, and unselfishness.

These asanas stimulate all glands in proper working order, mainly Vishudha and Manipura.

Ujjayi

This Pranayama exercise is to activate thyroid glands:

- Sit on your yoga mat in a meditation pose.
- Breathe in with the glottis (upper part of the throat) with a humming sound while keeping your mouth closed.
- Hold your breath and lower your head to touch your chin to your chest.
- Hold the air as long as you can.
- Lift your head up and close your right nostril with your finger, and exhale the air through the left.

Vajra asana

If you sit in vajra asana for 10 minutes after your dinner, it will improve your digestion and prevent constipation and gastric problems. It also strengthens the pelvic muscles and relieves knee and back *pain.*

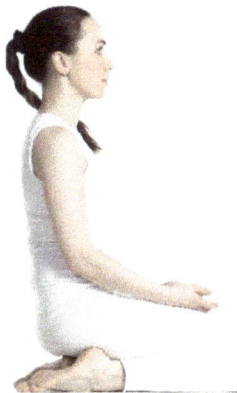

Mandukasana 1

- This pose is beneficial to all organs of the body.

- Mandukasana is very effective in diabetes, digestive disorders, and constipation.

- This pose improves the flexibility and mobility of the knee and ankle joints. (Ref: Swami Ramdev)

- It helps tone the muscles of the shoulder and abdomen.

- Regular practice of this pose increases your lung capacity.

- The frog pose helps reduce fat from thighs, belly, and hips.

- Sit in Vajrasana and make a fist while keeping your thumbs in; now join your fist together, make sure that your thumb side of the fist is towards the belly button.

- Press the fist to the belly button.

- Inhale

- Exhale by bending forward.

- Keep looking straight and hold your breath for a few seconds.

- Inhale and slowly back to vajra asana.

- Repeat 3 times.

Mandukasana 2

- Sit in Vajrasana and put your left palm at the navel or belly button and your right palm upon that.

- Inhale

- Exhale by bending forward.

- Keep looking straight and hold your breath for a few seconds.

- Inhale and slowly back to vajra asana.

- Repeat 3 times.

Balasana, the position of the child:

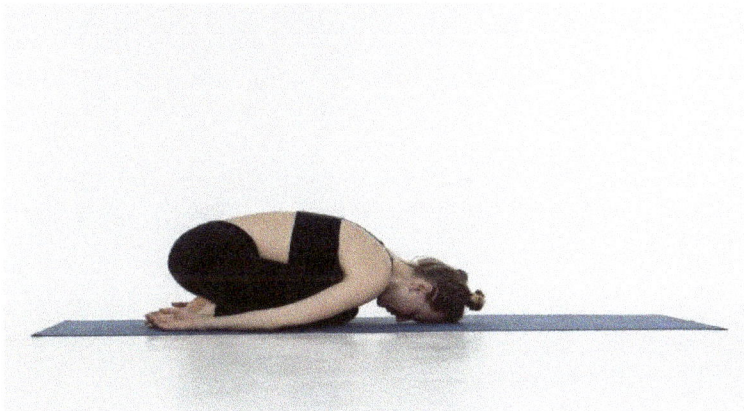

Through this position's daily practice, you can calm the mind, refresh the body, and eliminate the angry instinct. Flex your knees and bring your arms straight forward, rest your forehead on the mat and try to relax your neck and shoulders. Stretch your spine through the rhythm of your breath and relax your lower back

Pashimottanasana, the gripper posture:
You stretch the posterior thigh muscles, improve circulation throughout the spine, massage the internal organs, and release the accumulated anger and tension.

For Pashimottanasana, sit with your back straight, and your legs together and straight, and your toes face up. Then, with your spine upright and arms straight, move your hands toward your feet, go as far as you can; no need to give extra pressure or stretch to your body.

Padahastasana technique:

- Stand straight and tall with your feet and knees together. Keep hands at the sides.

- Lift hands above head while breathing in.

- Breath out, bend forward to touch the toes without bending the knees.

- Slowly, relaxing the lower back, squeeze the abdomen inwards and pull the torso forward so that the face touches the knee.

- Hold for 3-10 counts.

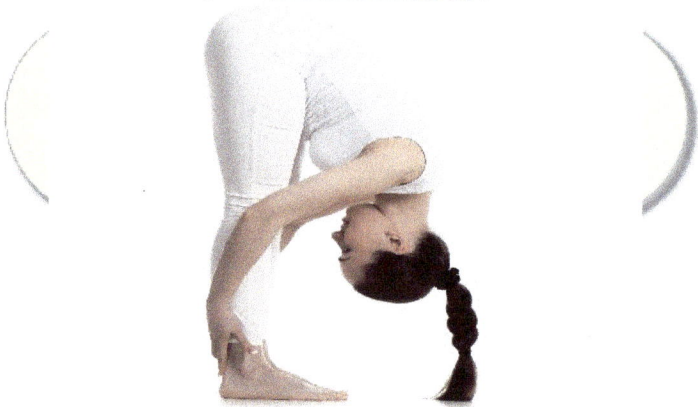

- Breathing in, come back up with hands above head

- Breathe out and drop hands to the sides.

The twisting postures are beneficial to overcome states of anger.

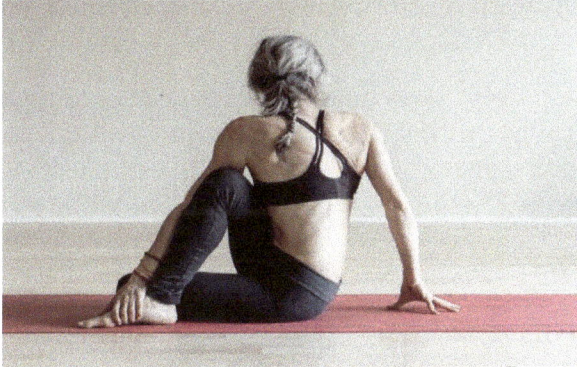

By rotating the trunk on one side and the pelvis, you can m a s s a g e the liver and look at the world from another perspective. You can perform the twist with your body lying on the floor or sitting with your legs crossed. When twisting, try to open your chest as much as possible, increasing the breadth of your breathing.

Savasana - The posture of the corpse.

Lie on the mat and relax your body. Bring your attention to your feet, then to your knees, pelvis, abdomen. Drop the wholebo shoulders, eyes, and every muscle in your face.

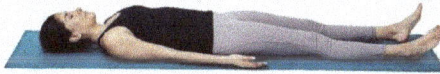

Breathing, the key to maintaining self-control

While practising yoga, try to meditate on the root of your anger; remember that it should not be repressed but metabolized in the present, here, and now. Each emotion requires deep attention and understanding to be overcome, which is why I advise you to watch it with detachment until you feel different.

Letting go of emotion means recognizing it to the point of preventing the feeling of identification with anger or frustration. The practice of yoga or oriental disciplines can be a valuable aid to restore balance.

Breathing control can help you deal with negative emotions. Focusing on breathing while doing the asanas, as mentioned above, will help you to improve self-control. Getting in the habit of doing these practices twice a day for just 3-5 minutes can yield long-term benefits.

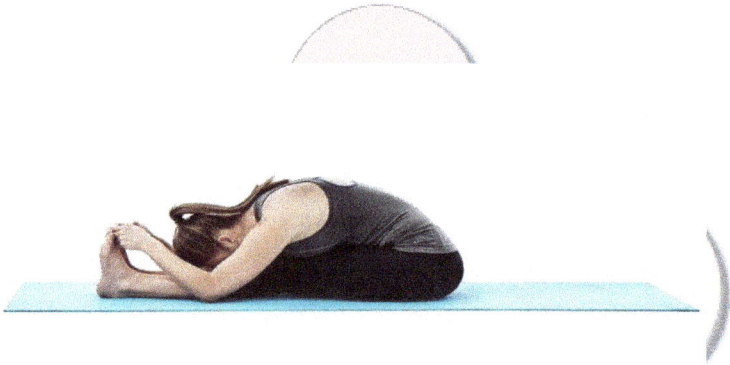

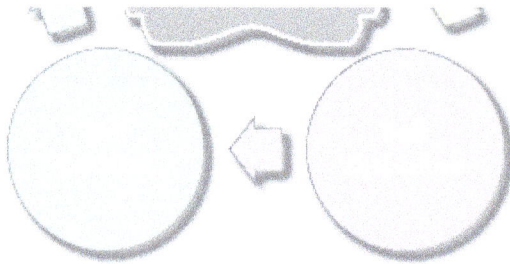

CHAPTER FOUR
Self-Motivation and Yoga

"First of all, it is established that no one will take my good mood away." The phrase of the writer Fernando Sabino translates well how the brain of a person with self-motivation. It is also an excellent incentive for those who are not feeling that excited.

Yes, while some complain about life, salary, the boss and even the time, the self-motivated remains calm and happy with their routine activities.

If the glass is half full, I can see that it is half empty or half full; it just depends on how you choose to see things. And the self-motivated naturally see things from a more positive angle. That is, for him, the glass will always be half full.

But how can we maintain a good mood and disposition amidst the countless daily tasks or adverse situations we face in our lives? Although it seems complicated, maintaining self-motivation is not an impossible task.

What is self-motivation?

Motivation is an incentive that comes from outside and helps us act. Self-motivation is the ability to motivate you without the need for any external factors.
And as we said in the paragraph above, developing self-motivation is possible (and we would also say precisely). But to do that, you need to be open to the new and willing to learn.

To learn how to self-motivate, you need to find out how you work, the best way to learn, how you feel in the face of the things around you, and, mainly, turn to yourself and take a little out of the focus of others.

This will help you understand what you want and focus on what matters.

Where is self-motivation born, that force so real and powerful that it makes us make extraordinary efforts to achieve our purposes? Where does this feeling of capacity come from? Our inner voice is responsible.

This voice, self-motivation, has the power to make us perform the most important daily actions, such as working, studying, walking etc. Our minds and thoughts are strong enough to give us enthusiasm and feed the passion we need to start our lives.

It is estimated that, on average, the mind processes 60,000 thoughts a day and around 40 thoughts per minute. We think and react accordingly. We live depending on countless emotional variables. Many of these thoughts go unnoticed, and we try to keep some that try to escape and others that, without realising it, become part of our reality.

We started to make opinions about ourselves and the space around us at a very young age. Opinions become ideas, judgments, or concepts that a person has or builds about something or someone.

Opinions are respectable; they come from the diversity of each individual. This does not mean that each opinion is true! Objectively, it is impossible to guess those 60,000 thoughts we talked about earlier. They are just personal judgments with no guarantee of validity. Many of these thoughts and opinions help to move forward and inspire and reflect our self-motivation. Others sabotage us by taking away our well-being, becoming factors that discourage us.

Tips to Maintain Self-Motivation

Be curious

Curious people are constantly chasing after something else. Mainly because curiosity challenges you to do things differently.

This is also an important feeling that takes us out of our comfort zone. And with that, it helps us to see the world in different ways. Being curious encourages us to seek solutions that no one else has seen, opening an immense universe of possibilities.

Allow yourself to change.

Take a risk regardless of the outcome. Be willing to grow and be open to new events, willing to be transformed by them.

Remember: planning is a means, not an end. So, more important than thinking about how you are going to accomplish something is doing it. Doing something keeps us excited, and that contentment fuels our self-motivation, no matter what the outcome.

That is, when it hits, the self-motivated celebrate, but the lesson learned from that situation is wrong.

Accept mistakes

If you want to maintain your self-motivation, persistencea n d resilience are words that should be very present in your vocabulary. Things that do not happen as you imagined should also be part of your routine.

It is important to note that: staying motivated is what will keep you going. So, keep thinking positive, but do not create too many expectations or false hopes about a situation.

Write down your goals (but get them off the paper!)

We all have short, medium, and long-term goals. But listing these goals in a list and marking them as soon as they are achieved encourages us to seek more results.

Not only that, having a plan for what we want (and what we have already accomplished) serves as a reminder and guide to show that attitudes have worked.

Writing your goals also helps in your organisation because it is easier to see what you need to do to achieve that goal by exposing your goals. This makes everyday tasks less stressful, as they will lead us to our ultimate goal.

Reward your earnings

More than being recognised by others, it is imperative that you recognise your achievements yourself. Thinking about it, how about rewarding each goal achieved?

Do not think about anything fancy but allow yourself something that gives you happiness. Go to the movies, have ice cream, sleep later, reward yourself in some way.

Many people tend to focus only on mistakes made, but successes can not only be celebrated but should be celebrated!

To have even more satisfaction in accomplishing something, create a hierarchy for your rewards according to the goals' importance. This will motivate you to stay focused until you reach your goal.

Do not worry; your brain will condition itself over time, and self-motivation will be naturally present in your daily life.

How to Stay Motivated by Doing Yoga at Home

Here are some tips to get that motivation how well it will do you:

- Just put on your yoga clothes. Those clothes that you are so comfortable in and make you feel like a Yogi.
- Start small. Maybe you want to start by sitting down to meditate or with some simple posture. Take your time, have an open mind. While doing yoga, a good trick is to think, "come on, just one more", instead of what you have left to finish.
- Take responsibility for your results. You can involve your partner or a good friend in your exercises; tell them that you are practising yoga and want them to be aware of it. If you do not like this option or do not think it is the best, you can write a diary of the days you have met or even write a blog. The idea that perhaps someone is reading how you are progressing in your practice or in your experience with yoga can be very motivating.
- Isolate your space to practice yoga. Put on a little of that zen music so that no noise distracts you. If you do not like doing yoga with music, you can try other things like – light a scented candle.
- Make space in your house. It does not take much. It can be the corner where you leave the bicycle or where you have placed that beautiful piece of furniture of your great- grandmother. You can sit in your garden in the fresh air if weather permits; otherwise, open the window to maintain airflow in the room. The important thing is that you can keep it simple and free from distractions. You can even make yourself an altar to practice yoga. Just have space where you can stretch out and unroll your mat. Give it a "holy" touch, at least in your mind.
- Set up a place in your life for yoga. Spend time and make your practice a priority. We know it is a lot easier said than done, but almost anyone can set aside 20-30 minutes a day, or at least a couple of times a week. Be flexible: early in the morning, after work or before going to bed, try it according

to your schedule. The more you practise, the more it becomes easier.

Using Yoga as a Motivator for a Better Life

Today, many yoga practitioners believe that the ancient discipline may serve as an incentive for individuals to relax and focus on what they want to accomplish in one way or another. It helps to pave the way to unite the breath, the mind, and the senses.

The word "yoga" refers to a Sanskrit term defined as "union or joining." This term has caused several people to be confused because it usually combines a range of purely physical to purely spiritual disciplines. The word 'asana' will never be left out when people talk about yoga. In comparison to physical stamina, asana poses are more focused on mental and spiritual well-being. Today, for modern practitioners of yoga, the two words have become almost synonymous with each other. This is because they symbolise the same notion that meditation is relaxation. Meditation in yoga can bring calm, mind calm, better health, better life, better relationships, personal insights, spiritual insights, philosophical insights, and a real sense of well-being.

Numerous studies have found that the musculoskeletal, nervous, endocrine and circulatory systems can be significantly affected by yoga. Therefore, this move will undoubtedly inspire one to live and appreciate the revitalisation of life.

While many people practise yoga for so many reasons, it serves as a motivation for people, especially those easily stressed out. One can explore the almost limitless possibilities of self-discovery by practising yoga. Yoga can indeed be a source of motivation for people who want the feeling of peace since its depths relate to meditative practice or pure spiritual discipline. People believed in Western cultures that gaps between the real bodies and the ideal bodies are increasing from time to time. This is due to the two main reasons for the lack of exercise and unhealthy diets that lead to heart problems, diabetes, and obesity. Thus, yoga is beneficial; it is all about experiencing pure ecstasy through the union of mind, body, and soul. While many yoga practitioners and teachers would agree that yoga can also serve as an incentive for people to have a better life, apart from providing relaxation and peace. This is because it gives a person unlimited opportunity to control and unite with the inner Self. This will thus create the balance that is needed in life.

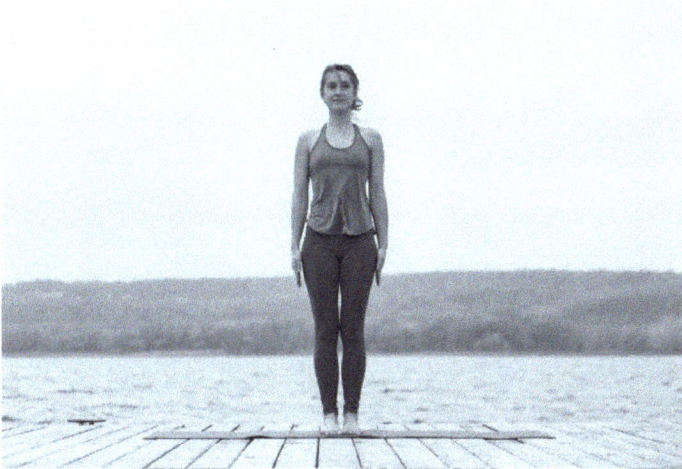

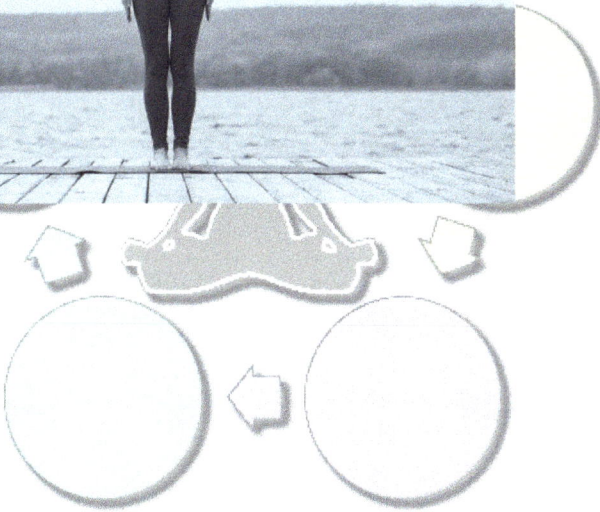

Yoga Poses for Confidence and Inner Strength

1. Tadasana

This asana will teach you how to maintain proper body posture.

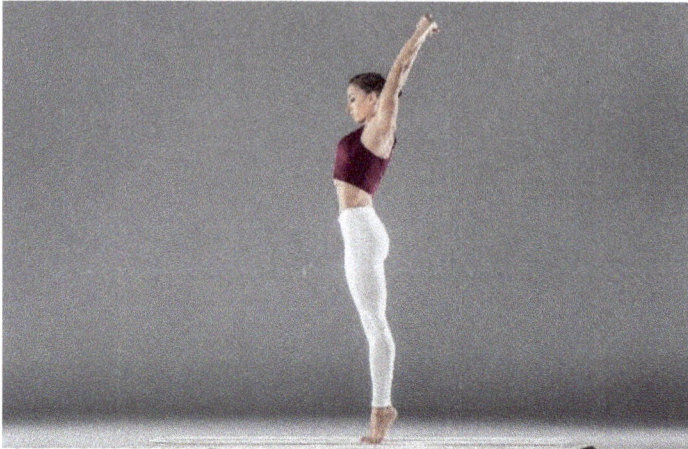

- Stand with your feet parallel, slightly apart. Feel the soles of your feet as the union of your being with the Earth. Feel your weight on them, make sure that your weight is balanced equally on both feet. Unlock your knees.
- Interlock your fingers, Inhale, raise your arms above your head with palms facing towards the ceiling.
- Stretch your body as much as you can on your tiptoes whilst keeping your back straight.
- The abdominal area should maintain a slight tension.
- Exhale and slowly back to your normal position by leaving the arms loose at the sides of the body.
- Repeat 3-5 times.

2. Virabhadrasana (Warrior Pose)

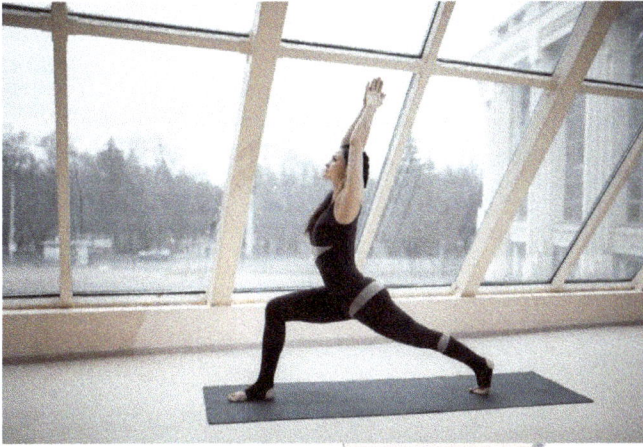

Being supported on your feet with your body's weight will give you the confidence you need to take firm steps.

- Stand straight and tall, put your right leg forward
- Maintain the posture and rest your heel flat on the floor. Correct posture - heels should be aligned.
- Ensure the right knee is in the same line as the heel of the right foot; besides, it must be bent at an angle of 90 degrees. If it is too flexed, it is an indication that you can spread your legs further apart.
- Face your right knee and bring your arms up. With each inhalation, feel your strength; With each exhale, go deeper into the pose.
- Repeat it on the other side.

3. Utkatasana (Chair pose)

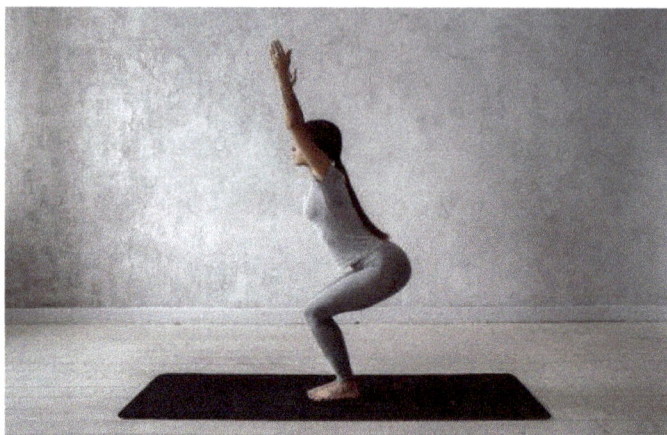

It is a posture that will help you gain control over your body and yourself. From the previous pose, bring your feet together at the front of the mat to begin this pose.

- Stand up straight, such as in tadasana or mountain pose, with your feet together this time.
- Raise your arms straight, with your palms together.
- Bring your hips back, like sitting in a chair. Keep your back straight.
- Try to stay in the pose for 10 breaths. To rest, return to the mountain pose.

4. Chaturanga dandasana (Four-Limbed Staff pose)

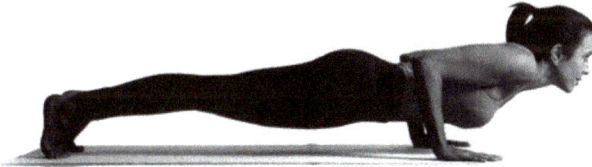

Drop forward from the mountain and move into this pose that will help you strengthen your body's core muscles.

- Place your hands on the sides of your chest. Bend your knees to support the palms of your hands.
- Make sure your hands are shoulder-length and flat on the floor.
- To move to the plank pose, slowly lift your body with your feet together.
- You are balancing your body on your elbows and toes. Your elbows should be bent at a 90-degree angle in plank pose, and your hands should be underneath.
- Try to hold the pose with your body straight for 10 breaths. To disarm, rest your knees on the floor and rest with your whole body face down.

5. Vasisthasana (side plank pose)

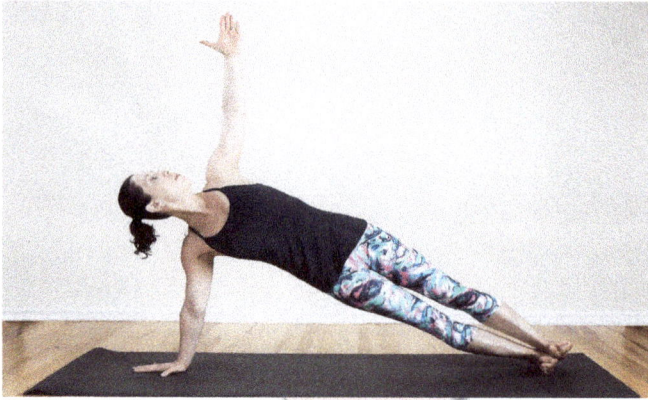

After you have rested, lie on your side on the mat and follow the instructions.

- Turn to one side, rest one of your elbows underyour shoulder and lift your body in a straight line.
- You can stay in this pose or lean on your hand to deepen the pose.
- The strength should be in your abs. This is the secret to keeping the body on one line.
- Repeat the pose on the other side.

6. Bhujangasana (Cobra pose)

It is a posture that makes you bring your shoulders back and open your chest to receive the energy of others while you plant yourself on the support of your hands and feet.

- Lie face down on the mat. Rest your hands on the floor below your shoulders.

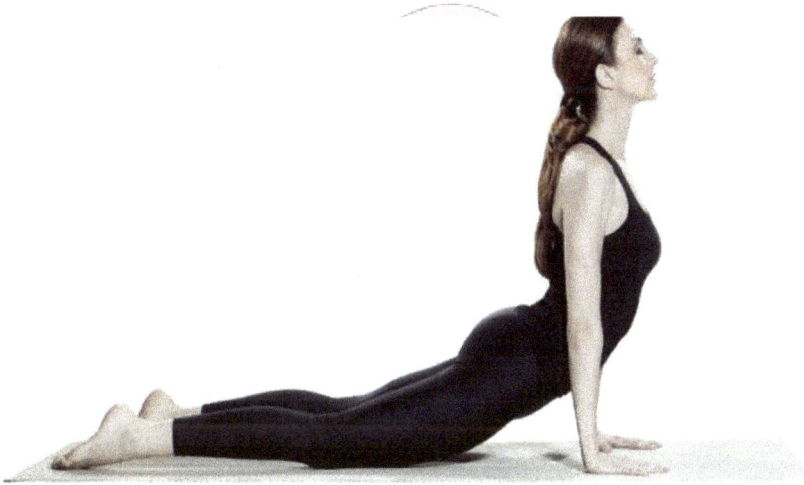

- Push yourself up with the strength of your arms. Let your whole body lift off the ground, except for your toes.
- Try to hold the pose for 10 slow breaths.

7. Ardha Chandrasana (Half Moon pose)

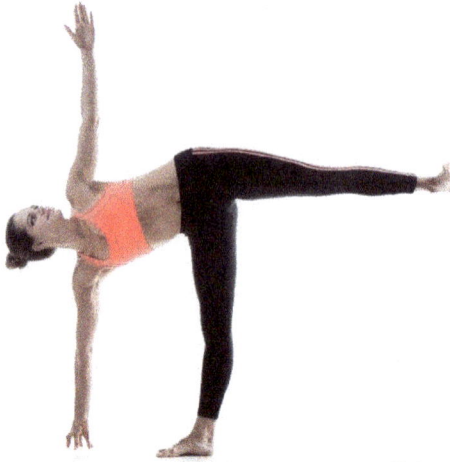

Nothing boostss e l f - esteem than setting a challenge with yourself, working for it, and sticking to it. For example, achieving a

- From mountain pose, lower yourself down and rest your fingertips on the ground in front of you. Keep your knees unlocked but your legs straight.
- Bring your right leg straight back.
- Begin to balance your left hand and left foot. This should be fully supported and on the hip line. The hand can rest on the ground, or you can support the fist or the fingertips, and even help you with a brick. The hand should be below the shoulder.
- When you are balanced, you can take your right hand off the floor and rotate your body to the side.
- Bring your right arm up, straight, and extend your right leg back.
- Hold the pose for 10 breaths and disarm it by slowly returning to all four supports. Rest before repeating it on the other side.

CHAPTER FIVE
Self-Healing and Yoga

Yoga has become one of the most recommended health specialists' methods; both doctors and psychologists advise their patients. People go to yoga classes for the most diverse reasons. Some need a bit of calm in their lives; others seek to relax and heal their bodies. Yoga is so rich and vast that when asked what it is for, it can be answered that it goes from healing to relaxation to enlightenment: how broad its spectrum is.

Although it expanded only a few decades ago in the West, the truth is that yoga is a method of self-knowledge and self-healing that humanity has practised for millennia. It implies the implicit perspective that we have the potential from which we can develop if we can unite and balance all the dimensions of our being. This means that we are both naturally multidimensional beings and have the possibility and the responsibility to become integral beings.

The mind, body and emotionality are aspects of the expression of our essential being. In a natural state, they are maintained in a state of balance and fluidity, in the form of health at all levels, expressing themselves in general harmonious functioning. This multidimensionality, then, means that each aspect of us is reflected in the other, empowering itself in the sense of growth or, if they are in shock or destruction.

It is essential to begin to improve our quality of life to know and recognise that we have within us a potential of enormous wealth: health, vitality, balance, strength, clarity. Through meditation, we reconnect with the deepest part of ourselves and then return all that internal potentiality to capacity.

Unfortunately, the context in which we were born and in which we move unfortunately does not help us achieve the latter. Instead, we are immersed in a culture that has been dedicated to fragmenting us for centuries.

The internal shock cuts off vital spontaneity, individual creativity, and the drive for self-expression. We feed erroneous beliefs about ourselves, about others, about our environment. We weaken, filling ourselves with guilt and fear. We become more irritable and eager for that lost fullness that we try to fill without external prostheses' success.

Somehow, we believe that by complying with all social mandates, creating a mask and hiding what happens to us, we can supplant our lack of love, meaning and internal cohesion. We can try our whole life.

Fragmentation and lack of love (of unity) are then what makes us sick. In shock and permanent isolation, the different aspects of ourselves easily enter a potentiated process in destroying our natural organism. Thus, weaken our immune system, allowing any negativity to nest in us. Stress, fear, anguish, which produces the state of internal division, wears us down, ages us, and stiffens us.

The result is that this energy that should naturally flow is blocked. And suddenly, we find it challenging to breathe physically, emotionally, and mentally.

It is necessary to repeat that we have all the potential and tools to live an entire life and become whole and self-aware beings.

It is at this point where practice comes in. As we said, yoga is a method for recovering the lost unity within ourselves and the Universe. The key here is in the experiential self-knowledge, learning and opening ourselves to feel.

The practice of meditation allows us this communication through deepening in the present state. It is essential to know that each person can start exercising from the place and state they are, regardless of age or condition. There is always the first step when starting anything.

The healing will begin with the reconnection with this natural state of which we spoke. At this point, it is worth clarifying that when we seek to heal, it is not something that we must add, but that health is something that we must recover. Nature is health in itself; it is fluidity and free expression. The disease arises when we block circulation, communication, and contact with this state. We alter

54

this course, forgetting our essence to identify ourselves with agitation, dialysing and attaching ourselves to passing states. Still, we substantiate our narrow gaze, fearful and ignorant of our great growth potential.

We will find that breathing is our greatest ally in practice, helping us maintain consciousness and connect with ourselves by achieving a state of attention and relaxation. We will experience that the deeper we breathe, the easier it will deepen the body and mind's union. That will gradually become more permanent.

The body helps the mind, and the mind helps the body simultaneously. We are a self-healing unit. A unit that can be sensitive, strong, and can maintain open attention free from distractions. In this way, we avoid wasting energy on unnecessary tensions and establish a naturally balanced and harmonic dynamic.

So, where does the healing force come from? Strength arises from ourselves when we unite the parts that previously worked separately. When we integrate mind, body, and emotions, overcoming the conflicts established between feelings, reason, imagination, and sensations. Instead of repressing, we open ourselves to knowing ourselves, understanding our vital needs, reconnecting with nature, and recovering the energy.

Yoga is an act of love. It re-connects our mind with our body by turning all that energy in our favour.

 It generates a strong axis with roots in our own hearts to understand ourselves and understand others.

When the balance is reestablished, self-confidence arises that allows us to overcome any problem, making fear dissolve. Stress dissipates. Calm will enable us to see everything clearly to make better decisions and not collapse in moments of crisis.

 Keep all fears, anguish, and anger in the shadows we use to grow in courage, self-esteem, compassion, and wisdom. We learn from what happens to us instead of martyrdom.

In this way, we become friends with ourselves and the same energy that previously damaged us start to heal us. It is the same energy;

it is the same mind, but with a change in attitude and perspective. We stop being in a defensive attitude to move to an active mindset. The clarity that practice allows us to develop the rechannelled force in the relaxation of unnecessary control makes us capable of discovering our evolutionary potential and making it a reality.

As we become more and more integral beings, we are returning with our nature and the Universal nature of our part, which nourish ourselves with clear consciousness.

The conscious human being exists. We carry it within. We only have to awaken our immanence to transcend our limits, converting all potential intelligence into realization.

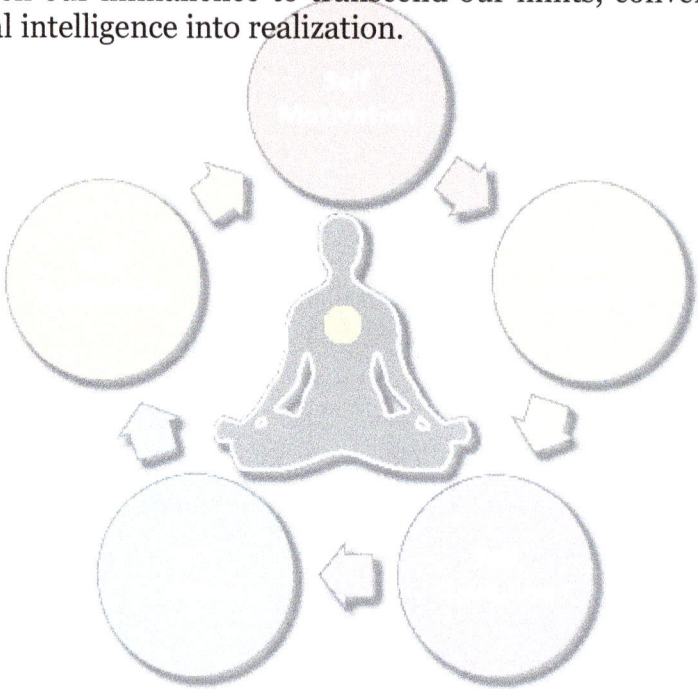

Self-Healing: The Power of Metaphysical Healing Techniques

Typically, individuals use it as a physical problem to treat illness or illnesses. This will be enough most of the time - there are excellent medications around the globe that can cure all kinds of issues.

However, healing requires more than just a physical type of healing. Metaphysical healing techniques address the fundamental problems leading to personal recovery.

Using these techniques, people can help themselves to prevent negative energies that can cause illness.

Here, we will introduce you to the top-recommended metaphysical techniques for healing.

- **Healing of your chakras**.
As I have explained, the importance of chakras in our life. The Chakra system exists within the subtle body, consisting of seven energy centres called chakras.

The chakras are responsible for regulating the flow of metaphysical energy through our bodies. For everything to go as it should, the chakras must be wide open so that the energies can enter accurately.

Those chakra's energies must be in balance with each other to prevent them from accumulating within one of the chakras on which they remain. Unfortunately, life can be complicated when it comes to those things.

You can also observe that most people's energy is stuck in two chakras – Muladhara and Manipura – sex and stomach. The flow of the energy should move freely to the top chakra (Sahastrara).

Certain Yogis exercises awakened the latent electric power and made it move upwards through different chakras. For example, when it goes up and penetrates through Muladhara chakra- sex glands, the sex power increases, when it penetrates Swadisthan chakra – Pancreas – adrenal, it improves digestion: when it penetrates Vishudha chakra, thyroid and parathyroid- it intensifies the process of purifying the body and tends to make it strong; when it penetrates Ajna Chakra- pituitary gland, one is able to command, and when it penetrates Sahatrar chakra- pineal gland, there is a light which can be seen in the middle of the forehead with closed eyes.

The Sahastrara (Pineal gland) acts as an organiser and controller of all glands. It controls the development of the glands and regulates them. The predominance of this gland generates a sense of sublimity- helping men and women grow into sainthood, endowed with divine qualities. These people have great wisdom and strong willpower and so are not affected by the body's sufferings or sorrow.

CHAKRAS INFORMATION

SAHASRARA	**CROWN** Connection of Godness, the Divine Source
AJNA	**THIRD EYE** Wisdom and spiritual awakening
VISHUDDHA	**THROAT** Creativity and communication
ANAHATA	**HEART** Love and kindness
MANIPURA	**SOLAR PLEXUS** Willpower and self-confidence
SVADHISTHANA	**SACRAL** Sexuality and sensuality
MULADHARA	**BASE** Sense of safety and grounding

Electricity reaches the brain. It slowly activates one by one 20,000 chips of our super computer, and a sense of new awakening-knowledge starts emerging from within. One gets a new perception of things, a new meaning of life.

Malfunctioning of this gland can cause serious problems, disturbing all other glands (chakras) proper functioning.

There may be negative energies blocking the flow. Remember that over stimulating the energy centre of one of the chakras over other chakras will lead to

You must practice meditation or promote energy flow through visualization, attention, and affirmations to heal your chakras.

Accupressure/ Reflexology

We should be grateful to those unknown sages/gurus who discovered the points to be pressed for treatment under this therapy installed in our palms and soles.

Our body is well equipped. Nature has provided in our body an "inbuilt mechanism". The health science which makes use of this inbuilt mechanism is popularly known as Acupressure". This therapy is the most exciting gift to mankind from the creator himself.

Acupressure therapy was known in India even 5000 years ago (Sushruta Samhita). Unfortunately, it was not preserved at that time and went to Ceylon in the form of acupuncture. From Ceylon, this therapy was taken to china and japan by Buddhist monks or nomadic aryas. At present, China is teaching acupuncture to the world. This therapy was known to Red Indians (nomadic Aryas who settled in the USA) way back in the sixteenth century. In the twentieth century, research has been done in the USA, significantly contributing to this therapy's development. World health organization has paid attention to this simple and easy therapy.

Acupressure is related to Acupuncture 'Acu' means needle, and to 'puncture' means to 'pierce'. So acupuncture implies the art of treating disease by piercing specific points in the body. Acupressure means the art of treating conditions by applying pressure on specific points with the help of one's thumb or unpointed things.

The concept of this therapy is based on the electric flow in our bodies. Our body's life battery flows the energy to maintain all systems work appropriately like an electric system in our homes. If any problem or default occurs in any connection, you will sense fluctuation means pain or uneasiness. If it is related to a specific area, you will get symptoms related to that particular area. The severe health issue considered a blockage of energy. The blocked flow of energy is the root cause of disease in people.

Fortunately, we have switches(points) in our palms and soles. Applying pressure on those switches can help release blocked energy and regulate the flow of energies within your body.

Despite apparent health benefits, these techniques will also provide metaphysical healing as they stimulate energy flow. You can check all your pressure points in palms and soles on google.

The best thing I told my group is that when you apply the cream before bed on your hands and feet, massage your palms and soles and press all over. Then, if you feel pain anywhere, press that point for **at least 2-3 minutes**. You do not need to remember all the points; just massage and press all the points regularly.

- **Appreciate yourself.**

This is the most straightforward metaphysical healing technique known to humans, and it is called human kindness.

Science showed that loving yourself improved patients' chances of recovery.

Your mind is a mighty thing. Your mind is the one that controls your whole body.

Therefore, you must practice kindness to yourself every time you wake up. A little acceptance and self-love can go a long way when it comes to getting rid of the negative energies that are constantly dragging you down.

Yoga for Emotional Healing

Like so many other things, emotional health is typically considered only when it has reached a point where it is out of balance. We are still mostly negligent concerning emotional health and well-being in such a modern culture. Many of us are willing to pay attention to our feelings only when they have become a serious issue.

Fortunately, modern society has a more significant personal role to play in their well-being and health. But, unfortunately, because of the prevalent belief that emotional problems are a sign of weakness within our minds, we do not seek the correct emotional health information.

The need for emotional healing can manifest itself as something large, such as an emotional breakdown or crisis, or as small and unassuming as a sense of unease or dread underlying it. We tend to toss ourselves into distraction when the symptoms are mild. These distraction cycles keep our attention diverted for a while elsewhere, but the emotional turmoil is not gone; it is often only temporarily masked. This is how it can transform a small emotional disturbance into an all-out crisis.

If you wish to know the true state of your emotional health, look for any areas of excess in your life. Observe, but do not judge yourself.

The daily practice of yoga, for some reason, provides emotional healing and support. It is thought that the ego is a significant player in creating emotional disturbances in Yogic philosophy because it draws all conscious attention to itself. During a daily Yoga session, conscious awareness is diverted from the ego, and true emotion can be felt in those moments. It is very healing - in and of itself   - to turn conscious attention towards   one's true emotions. An objective look at reality is very often all that is needed to encourage an internal and lasting change.

The emotional energy may still be felt through the physical body for some individuals who can no longer feel their emotions. For people who have survived great emotional turmoil and distressing situations because the emotions were disconnected from surviving, this seems to be a problem.

Rational people still have their emotions, but the emotions have been buried alive, deep inside the mind somewhere. Counselling is strongly recommended on the path of recovery for these individuals. Pranayama yoga can be used as a tool for self-healing.

It is believed that when individual moves through the asanas with breathing control, the conscious mind then becomes aware of the emotion, and feeling may be turned toward the focus. As part of everything, it can then be accepted, releasing the system's emotion. The moment emotional baggage buried comes into conscious awareness, it will start to disappear in meaning, bringing the conscious state of mind into balance.

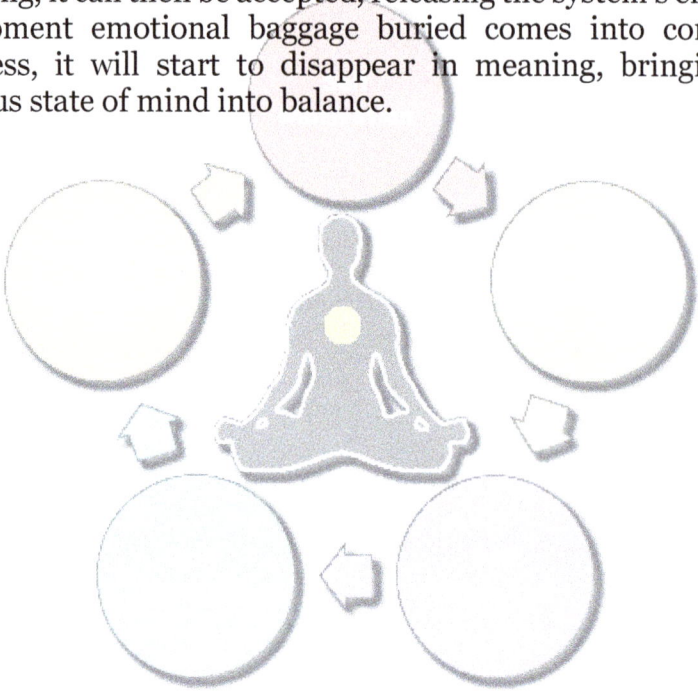

Yoga Poses for Self-Healing:

1.Surya Namaskar (salutation to sun)-

Surya Namaskar is a practice of Yoga that is traditionally performed to warm up more challenging poses. The sun is the source of life on earth. Therefore, these ancient yogis believed that worshipping the sun would lead to good health.

Surya Namaskar is a way to say hello to the sun, a source of the universe's energy and lifeline. It is the best way to start your day. It is known as a full-body stretch. It unwinds the mind and body. It should be done in the morning, facing the sun (direction east) to benefit Surya Namaskar.

It strengthens your neck, shoulders, arms, wrists, finger, abdomen, intestine, thigh, knees, calves, ankles, and most importantly, core and back.

If we talk about benefits, there is a long list; the main possible benefits are:

Improves energy level

Boosts immunity

Enhances physical strength Improves digestion

Reduces fat around the abdomen

Makes the spine and waist more flexible

Make the heart and lungs stronger.

Remove tensions of your muscles

A secret of beautiful skin.

Improves blood circulation in the body and

Improve concentration.

It is a set of 12 asanas known as complete body stretching and exercise. If you do around 20-25 sets in the day, that means you are done for the day.

How To Make Surya Namaskar - A Step By Step Process

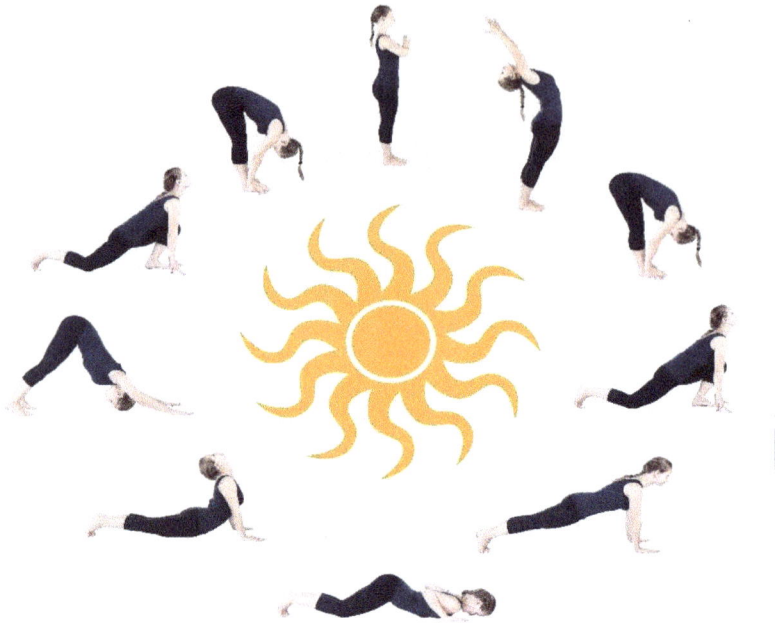

Here is a detailed breakdown of the Surya Namaskar steps for anyone wondering how to do Surya Namaskar at home.

1. Pranamasana (Prayer posture)

Put your feet together and balance your weight on your feet equally. Next, expand your chest, and as you inhale, raise your arms on both sides, bring them together in front of the chest in the prayer position as you exhale.

2. Hasta Uttanasana (Raised arms pose)

Then inhale again and, with your biceps close to your ears, raise your arms up and back. Ensure that your entire body is stretched from your heels to your fingertips.

3. Hastapadasana (Standing forward bend)

Lean forward with your spine erect as you exhale and lower your hands to the ground next to your feet.

4. Ashwa Sanchalanasana (Lunge Pose)

Push your right leg back as far as possible while you inhale. Look up then and bring your right knee down to the ground.

5. Chaturanga Dandasana (Plank Pose)

Similarly, with your body in a straight line and your arms perpendicular to the floor, take your left leg back as you inhale and go to the plank position.

6. Ashtanga Namaskar (Eight Limbed Pose)

Exhale and lie down with your knees together. Then bend your knees slightly and put them together. Raise your back slightly; eight points on the body - two hands, two feet, two knees, chest, and chin - should be the only points of contact between your body and the floor.

7. Bhujangasana (Cobra Pose)

Lift your chest with your elbows bent and your shoulder away from your ears. Stretch out as much as possible and make sure your chest pushes forward when you inhale. When you exhale, push your navel down gently.

8. Adho Mukha Svanasana (Downward-Facing Dog)

Lift your hips and tailbone with your palms still on the floor so that your body forms an inverted "V" shape. Make sure your heels touch the ground so your body remains straight.

9. Ashwa Sanchalanasana (Lunge Pose)

The inverted V returns to an equestrian stance with the right leg back and the chin facing up in one fluid motion. Stretch your body as much as possible.

10. Hastapadasana (Standing Forward Bend)

You should turn your legs' end and make them perpendicular with your hands by placing your hands on the floor above them.

11. Hasta Uttanasana (Raised Arms Pose)

Continuing the reverse trend, extend your spine as you exhale and raise your hands above your head. Stretch more instead of reaching back.

12. Pranamasana (Prayer Pose)

Exhale slowly, lower your arms and back to namaskar mudra and Relax and observe the various sensations that run through your body.

2. Long Holds: learning to feel

When we hold postures for a long time, our feelings begin to bubble up. As we focus on the inside, we become more aware of what is happening.

Holding poses activates our feelings and emotions. We started listening, and we feel what is coming. We will notice that postures have more tension than others. They are likely to be the same ones that will heal most.

Pose: Mandukasana (Frog Pose)

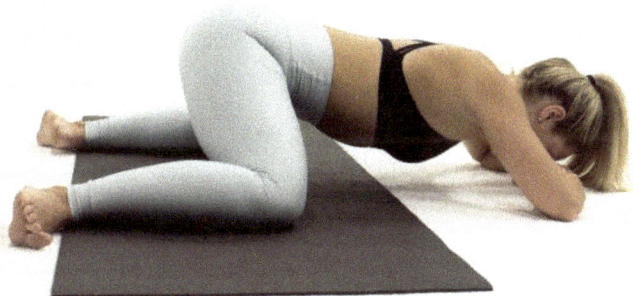

This pose can become very

ıe breath at a time. It is important to note that discomfort and pain are two different things: try to go through the discomfort; get out of the pose if you feel any pain.

3. Grounding: the mind-body connection

The first step in reducing current trauma is to establish a strong connection in mind to the body. To be healed, one must learn to look to within.

We can touch our bodies through yoga because it forces us to check in with our physical sensations. The more we practise observing our thoughts as they arise, notice more emotions springing up to the surface.

Grounding practise is a great way to form a powerful mind-body connection because you are both supported by the ground and in your body at the same time. The Recliners allow us to feel and be held simultaneously.

Pose: *Supta Baddha Konasana (Bound Angle Reclining Pose)*

Supta Baddha Konasana is good to do while fully relaxing on the mat. Place one hand on your heart and one hand on your belly to keep your attention on your breathing and the present moment.

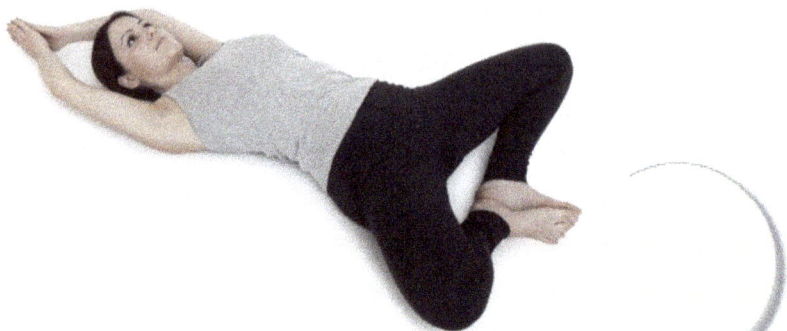

4. Surrender: Emotional release

Sometimes all we need to heal is letting go. But, unfortunately, letting go has become a cliché in yoga bubbles.

However, letting go does not necessarily mean releasing the pain or anger; sometimes, it means surrendering to it; letting go of it.

Often, we resist feelings that do not feel "right." But, feelings are neither good nor bad. They are what they are. It is our resistance to the feeling that causes us pain.

So sometimes, we just must give in to our feelings to heal them completely.

Pose: Eka Pada Rajakapotasana (Half Pigeon Pose)

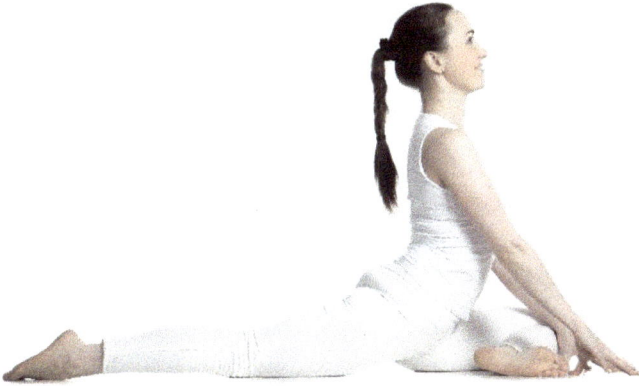

Pigeon Pose is a great place to come up with some creativity. Unfortunately, because of all the emotions that occur at our hips, we often have no choice but to give up after slowly opening our hips deeply.

A pigeon is perhaps a place that brings tears frequently, and those are completely normal emotions. However, by staying here, we can break through the walls that we have surrounding past experiences. When we do this, we often bring about emotional release and negative feelings. This makes it very healing.

5. Heart Openers: Vulnerability

Have you ever had that instance in the class where you experienced a 'light bulb moment'? As a recognition, you are beginning to understand why you have felt this way for many years.

Yoga teaches us to be very open and vulnerable to our feelings. Vulnerability is a precious part of our healing. When we cannot be vulnerable, we begin to pare down our relationships. We give ourselves physical and mental "protection" by building walls around our hearts, making us more vulnerable to harm.

We must open our hearts to find love for ourselves, heal our wounds, and love others completely.

The heart's opening and closing motions also allow the blood to expand and relax. As spiritual beings, we open the vaults inside full of a charged energy by opening our hearts to others.

Pose: Urdhva Dhanurasana (Wheel Pose)

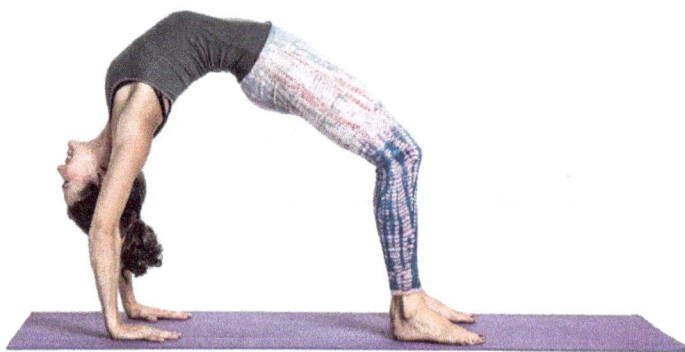

The wheel is a deep heart opener that helps us tear down those walls and learn to open our hearts.

This is an excellent pose because we open our hearts, but we have our hands and feet on the ground while keeping us grounded.

6. Balance: Responding vs Reacting

Very often, when we get angry, we react rather than appropriately respond. Memories can turn into regrets. When we snap, we do not take a moment to think or even get a second to breathe before speaking and ending up hurting someone else or ourselves.

Yoga can help one learn how to respond to tense or unfortunate situations with an equal mind attitude. Instead of the general effect of the situation, the more direct response results in a calmer and more friendly interaction. We should react to this situation to walk away, feeling much better than being frustrated and reacting negatively.

Pose: Natarajasana (Dancer Pose)

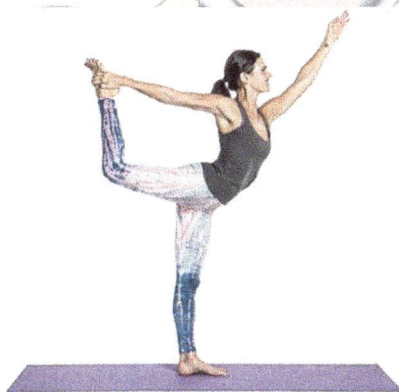

Balance poses help us learn how to respond. For example, when we fall from a balancing pose, like a Dancer, we have two options: we can get angry and frustrated that we failed, or we can take a deep breath, maybe even smile, and do it again.

7. Self-empowerment: Courage

Finally, we must bring our inner power to life to heal past traumas. This is not power that is aggressive or controlled; it is empowerment. It is confidence, courage, truth; It is a willingness to appear in your life.

Self-empowerment is a place where you recognise your path and do not run away from it. Instead, you embrace it. And you embrace all that you are: strengths and flaws alike.

Pose: Virabhadrasana II (Warrior 2)

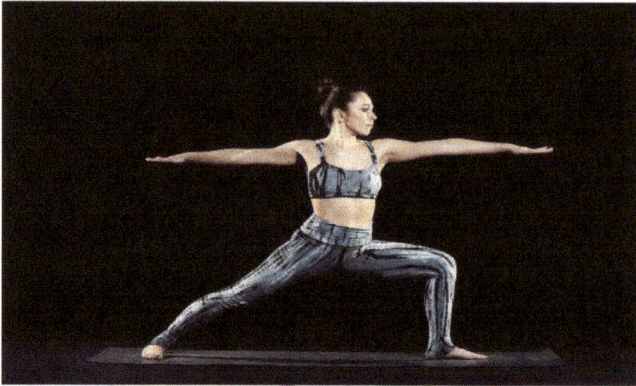

Warrior 2 helps us dive deep into our power. Create a fire in our legs and a feeling of freedom in our hearts.

Let yourself be amused by this pose. Play with arm variations and stick around a little longer than you would like. You will be surprised at what comes inside.

Yoga can help you cure headaches and trauma just as much as it can enhance flexibility and strength. But you must enter with an open mind and heart, approach your mat. Do this, and there will be healing. Slow but secure.

8. Ahinsa: Non-violence

Ahinsa translates to' non-violence' from Sanskrit. Therefore, the concept that all living things are sacred should not be harmed is inspired by it.

This applies to you as well. We talk about being nice to others a lot, but we forget about ourselves sometimes. We should treat each other similarly, just as we should treat others with kindness and compassion.

A lot of us tend to be tough on ourselves. Whether it is the way we look, how smart we are, or our general position in life. Think about how when you make a mistake, you talk to yourself. Yoga teaches us that we should be gentle with ourselves. When we need to listen to our body. Slowly, when we are tuned in with our feelings and emotions, we learn how to heal ourselves.

Pose: Balasana (Child's Pose)

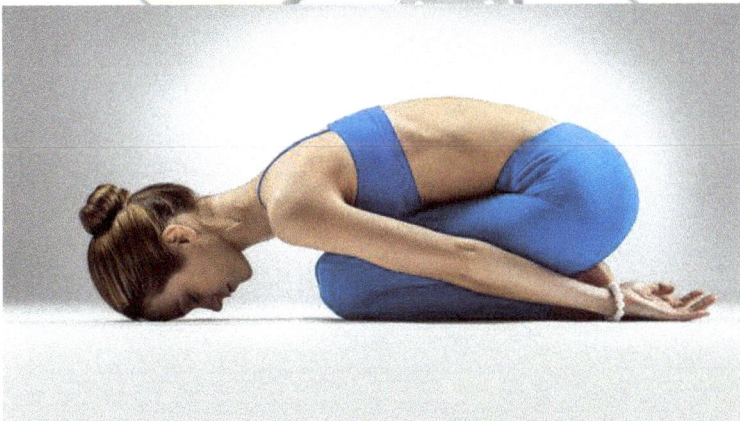

Oftenall it takes is areturn to basics. The child's posture serves many purposes, one of which is as a resting place.

Take the child's pose in class every time your body tells you to slow down. You can even take it on its own whenever you feel overwhelmed.

9.Relaxing:

The first step of learning Savasana is to learn how to breathe deeply and slowly. When stressed, people usually breathe shallow and fast. Sometimes they hold their breath when they feel stressed and are not even aware that they are doing it.

Research shows that Savasana:

1. Relaxes and calms the body

2. Increase the focus of mind and concentration

3. Improves blood circulation and lower blood pressure 4. Relief from headache and improve sleep

5. Improve the heart's rhythm

6. Increase blood circulation

7. Sharpen mental performance

8. Helps to reduce back pain

Before you start trying to do Savasana, it can be helpful to try noticing how you are breathing: Lie down on your back, put one hand on your stomach and the other on your chest. Notice the movement of your hand as you breathe.

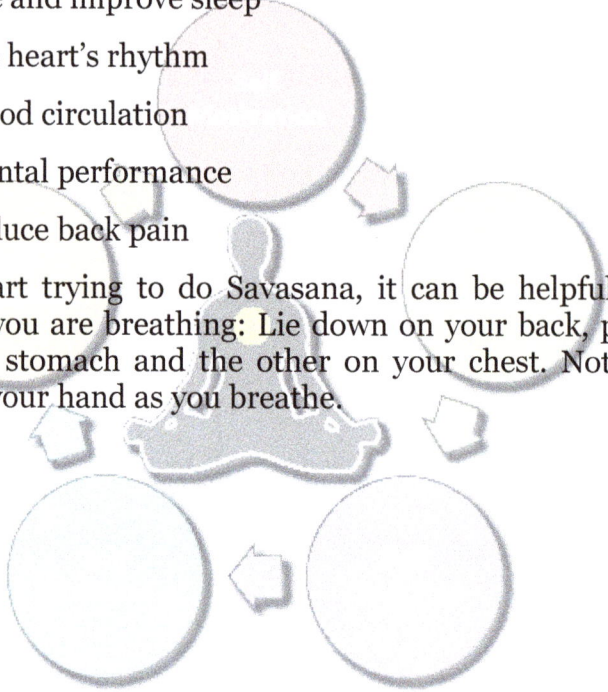

Pose: Savasana (Corpse Pose):

- Lie down on your mat in a comfortable position with hands open at sides and legs wide open (as much as you feel comfortable).
- Mark a point at the ceiling and stare at that point, deep breath in and out.
- Count 10 to 1 while breathing deep.
- On 1 close your eyes, relax your body
- Try to focus on each part of the body, starting with toes to the top of the head and brain.
- This process will relax and rejuvenate your whole body. You can try when you are tired or exhausted; it will fill you with fresh energy.

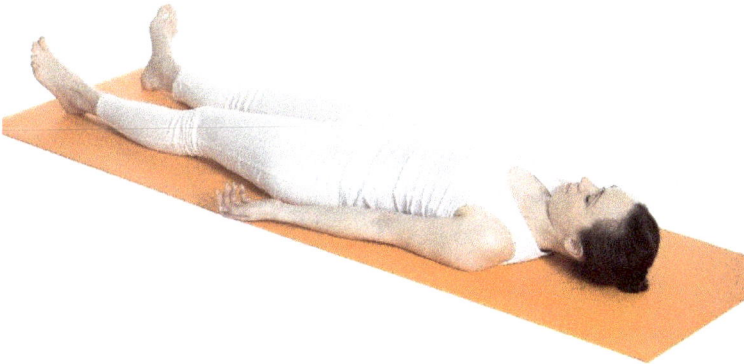

CHAPTER SIX

Self-Realisation and Yoga

Self-realisation is a translation of the term atmasakshat Kar from Sanskrit. The literal translation is "the manifestation of your spirit." This is a spiritual transformation of a person, which allows him to connect with the Absolute energy. This union (union, yoga) is carried out by the Chakras energy. This is the most important chakra, sitting at the top of the head "Sahastrar". When we reach this chakra. We can experience the opening of a third eye – a sense of sublimity.

Self-realisation is not a mental process, not hypnosis or self-hypnosis. You can feel it as a cool breeze overhead and on your arms.

Why is this needed, and what does it give?

Self-realisation is your right, which belongs to you from birth. Whether to use it or not is up to you. Self-realisation gives knowledge about the subtle energy system within you. This knowledge is not bookish, not abstract, not emotional. You will be able to feel the state of each chakra at your fingertips and determine what you need to do to improve yourself. Having received self-realisation, you gain knowledge about your chakras. This knowledge will allow you to prevent at an early stage of the disease (since the disease first manifests itself in the form of negativity in the chakras). For this, there are simple methods of cleansing the chakras.

Steps to Achieve Self-Realisation

Self-realisation is one of those words whose meaning varies greatly depending on each individual. However, we can describe it in simple terms. It is a psychological state of euphoria or complete happiness due to previous actions and decisions that we have made in life. We can trace the origin of this way of thinking to the philosopher Aristotle, who said that there are two virtues necessary to achieve this state of mind: intelligence and character. We can also link the concept of self-realisation to Eastern religion as a spiritual state of "self-knowledge.

Are we pursuing self-realisation in your life? Well, yes, in one way or another, all of us would like to experience a deep sense of satisfaction in having had a worthwhile existence. However, what is the reasons that make our life worthwhile? Although people have different motivations to be happy, we must explore some that exist that are distinct aspects for all of us as human beings:

- Goals:

Of course, our desires vary widely: some people are driven by money or power, other people want athletics, musical talent, academic prowess, true love ... but what links us to us is that we all form goals in our brain as a means of obtaining our wishes. In this way, we have an idea of what we want to achieve and how we will do it. The benefit of having specific purposes is motivation and ambition that we feel to fulfil them. However, these goals must also be challenges that are outside of our element. We will never get true satisfaction from self-realisation if it is something very easy to obtain. Similarly, they must be realistic and achievable to avoid a sense of disappointment if they are not met.

- Learning:

Another useful element to achieve self-realisation is to study to have a clearer point of view of the world which complies with "the virtue of intelligence" and "the knowledge of oneself". These can be the lessons of mistakes and previous actions, or generally, they can be studies or training in a particular educational field. With learning first, we will have more opportunity to fulfil our personal goals. Greater knowledge means that we can help other people and help ourselves since we can react better as more informed individuals in the face of problems and difficulties. That is why we feel the sensation of personal well – being

- Socialisation:

It is essential to pursue goals and focus on progressing as individuals. At the same time, there needs to be a balance between career goals or personal dreams and fulfil social needs. According to Maslow's hierarchy of needs, we have a mutual need to interact with other people. Although this model is old-fashioned and rigid, the feelings of love and friendship are precious and essential in our lives. How can we fully appreciate any success without the reassurance and comfort of knowing that we are loved by family, friends, partners, etc.? These emotions give us self-esteem to reach our goals, and we can share our success with loved ones.

- **Acceptance:**

Ultimately, we need to accept that we have flaws and abilities, and perfection is impossible to progress. However, the truth is that a perfectionist will find it more challenging to achieve self-actualisation than a person who recognises his mental and physical strengths and weaknesses.

The perfectionist cannot accept his limits. If we can feel at peace with what we can achieve, then the key is to look at our strengths and develop them to the highest level.

In summary, although all these aspects are indeed applicable to everyone, it is also necessary to consider that everyone is at a completely different starting point searching for this joy. Quality of life, social and political environments, physical and mental well-being are examples of aspects that can facilitate or impede self-realisation. We can only get on with our lives in the hope that we achieve this intangible euphoria.

Get Your Self-Realisation!

The first thing you must do is decide if you want to get self-realisation. Getting self-realisation is voluntary; you cannot force anyone to do it. To obtain self-realisation (awakening of the Kundalini energy), choose 10-15 minutes during which no one can bother you. It is advisable to take off your shoes, watches, glasses and loosen all tight belts and buckles. Sit comfortably, relax, do not cross your legs, and place them at some distance from each other (these are different energy channels). Try not to remember any troubles, not to think about your past mistakes or inappropriate actions. Now, none of these matters; God forgives you unconditionally.

78

To Achieve this "S" (Self-realisation), we need to open to the universe. Sit in meditation by placing the left hand on the left knee and the right hand on the right knee. This symbolises your desire to receive Self-realisation.

Paths of Self-Realisation

The path to self-realisation ends at a single point: the self-understood consciousness as Atman, the Self without exception, all the self-knowledge paths end in the consciousness.

There are three main trails to reach a good port on this unique journey, which are not uncommon. The first consists of knowing that such a possibility exists, and then the theory of classical and sacred texts is resorted to, and some sacred rituals and activities.

Now you know that the possibility exists and just a few steps away from you to embrace it. If you are not able to reach to those steps; choose the second trail.

The next path is to follow the person who has the direct experience, who lives in such a state. He transmits you through their presence, turning on the light of consciousness, leading to direct teaching.

Finally, it proceeds through the daily practice of a Sadhana or spiritual path to protect and increase it until it lights the inner fire.

Over time, gentle perseverance, and installed in the Self, the Atman, comes the clear understanding that gives rise to wisdom, a characteristic feature of the self-realised being. It will undoubtedly happen with such premises because it is not something to be achieved but instead to allow it to happen.

People feel different after coming back from yoga retreat centres because they follow all steps like - open to receive, sitting religiously to receive and being influenced or motivated by the company of great yogis or practitioners.

Yoga, the best help

Why is yoga discovered as such a helpful instrument in the process of self-realisation? Because in no other science - we remember that yoga is the soul's science - are these three factors found together. On the one hand, Tradition and its literature speak to us about the real possibility of self-realisation —it is no utopia—, covering the area of theory.

On the other hand, it is possible to find self-realised beings who live in such a state of authenticity that their mere presence is enough to understand without words. Thus, the light of your consciousness has become a reference beacon to illuminate the shadows of Avidya, ignorance, turning them into Vidya, knowledge.

Finally, what is perhaps most important: Abhyasa, continuous practice. Such practice arises from the fruit of a sincere desire for authenticity born in the essence that inhabits every human being's interior. Practice, and not just reading books or attending Satsangs, is a great enhancer so that the journey of self-knowledge, of self-discovery, can come to fruition.

After all, self-realisation is not an impossible fantasy to achieve since a self-realised being has found what is Real in him. But, alas, human beings like to dissipate their energies and possibilities in fleeting trifles, rather than trying to discover who or what they are, with the potential that it entails.

Asanas That Bring You Closer to Self-Realisation

Asanas benefit all the body's systems: endocrine, respiratory, circulatory, nervous, and digestive. In yoga class, each posture is usually worked so that it stimulates and favours each area. As a result, you begin to feel that mind-body integration flows more naturally with just a few months of practice.

When you process more complex asanas, you give in to the nervous system, find peace in the emotions, and achieve a more profound and more restorative relaxation.

The most straightforward techniques of this discipline are those that use static physical positions. However, if you want to promote self-knowledge, dynamic postures, keep your mind focused on balance and movements. When asanas are static, mental functions are enhanced, and emotions are balanced.

Back bending poses

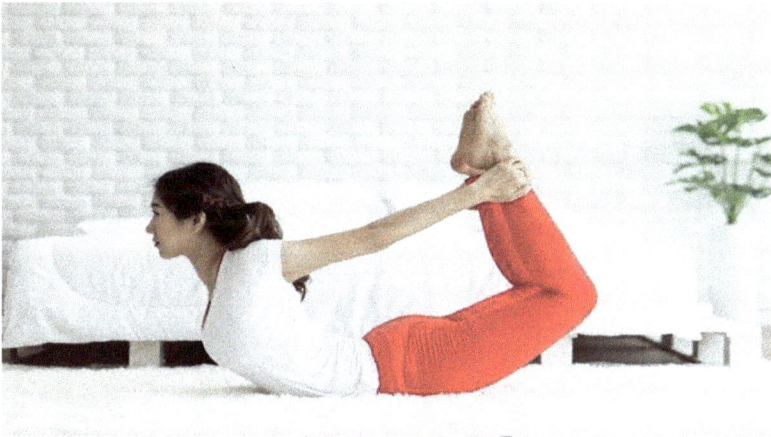

If you practice this ancient discipline, you know that each posture is related to another. Far from counteracting the benefits between one and the other, asanas' regular and balanced practice improves physical and mental capacities. The cobra, kidney massage and camel asanas are ideal if you are seeking self-realisation. These postures promote brain function, tone the spinal cord and spinal nerves. Most of the backward bending postures induce a feeling of expansion, while the forward bending positions lead us to personal recollection.

To these asanas, you can add the meditation ones at the end of a session. The technique of visualisation, during meditation, helps us explore our interior. The way you immerse yourself in it is the key to achieving objectives and goals.

Camel pose

This asana is done twice, about thirty seconds each. It has a score of benefits, including strengthening the back and pectoral muscles. In addition, provide elasticity to the spine and energise the brain.

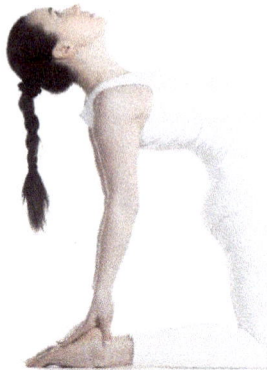

Cobra pose

It is a doubly beneficial asana for women because, in addition to revitalising the brain, it favours the ovaries and stabilises menstrual cycles. Moreover, it is a very applied position to combat mental dispersion and increase concentration. The time to maintain the posture is 30 seconds, a pause of a similar time and repetition of this asana.

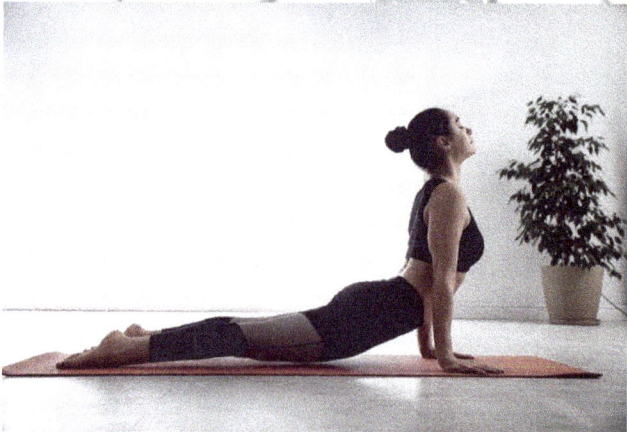

Kidney massage posture

Suppose you are looking to advance on your introspection path, overcome traumas, fears, and encourage yourself to forgive. In that case, this asana helps the feeling of physical and mental openness.

Unlocks and relaxes, as well as improves mental operations. This asana has a variant with a little more complexity. It is about bending the legs, as much as possible, and bringing the heels to the buttocks. Two asanas of 50 seconds each are performed.

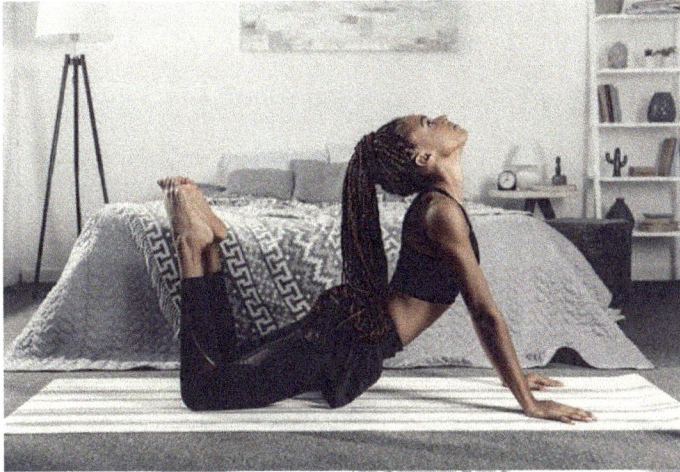

Physical and mental balance

When your body and mind come together for the same purpose, you are already working on personal fulfilment. The regular practice of this discipline makes you exceed your limits. When you start yoga, you learn about 30 basic postures that do not usually present much difficulty.

Therefore, each new asana you learn and perform successfully contributes to your satisfaction. However, only you know how much time and effort it has cost you.

We mentioned different types of posture related to all "S". However, all come closer the more you internalise this discipline. The personal growth that the most complex asanas provide is not in the goal achieved, but you have carried out to achieve it in the process.

CHAPTER SEVEN
Pranayama
Benefits and Techniques of Yogic Breathing

As I mentioned earlier in this book, the pranayama is the set of breathing techniques framed in practising yoga.

The purpose is to control what the Tradition of Yoga called prana in Sanskrit and referring to as cosmic energy. Several Pranayama techniques have been taught for millennia.

Asana and Pranayam are the 3 & 4 stages of yoga. They harmonize each other. They are interwoven together for better results. This combination is used in different types of Yoga techniques. But we will talk about pranayama yoga with the combination of gentle exercise, which will enhance you in all aspects of your life and lighten you to achieve all Self "S" for magnetic connection to the universe.

There are three types of breathing, abdominal, thoracic, and clavicular breathing. When they are all brought together effectively, we speak of complete breathing.

Pranayama techniques are how breathing is trained and are divided into significant and minor Pranayama techniques

Pranayama Benefits

The pranayama, or techniques to learn to breathe correctly, has many benefits (could not be otherwise, since there are many Yoga benefits). Some of them are:

- Increases lung capacity by taking a deep breath in and out.
- You have more stamina to perform physical efforts. Observe people who breathe badly. They tire quickly with little effort, such as walking up a flight of stairs.

- Generates tranquillity and peace of mind. Slow and sufficient breathing is the body's natural state, without tension, which also causes fatigue and mental fatigue.
- Revitalises the body. After exercising, you regain a normal heart and breathing rate. For what is this? Because you need less air than you have been using. Therefore, if your lung capacity increases, you feel better and more willing to move, go out for a walk, do physical exercise, etc.
- Slow, deep breathing reduces the heart's strain, which becomes more efficient and robust, works better, and lasts longer.
- In a moment of stress or anxiety, it manages to reduce it considerably and even eliminate it.
- If you are nervous, you can control your emotions and make the right decision without reaching a higher level of feeling stressed.
- Deep, slow breathing is an excellent weight regulator. If you want to lose weight, be aware that having higher oxygen levels in your blood helps you burn fat.
- It helps the body regain a normal rhythm after making some effort, physical or mental, in which there has been wear.
- It helps to sleep well since it calms the mind. However, the leading cause of insomnia is not knowing how to relax and putting problems aside until you have rested.
- Improves digestion. The body assimilates food better thanks to the greater oxygenation of the blood makes the digestion process more efficient.
- It is great for the skin. This is because the body directs most of the oxygen to the brain. Once that function is covered, the rest is distributed. Therefore, more oxygen is destined to the pituitary and pineal glands with better oxygenation, which are very important in skin rejuvenation.
- Induce the state of meditation.

Pranayama Yoga

According to Indian philosophy, our life is fixed and measured not by years but by the total number of breaths we take. Therefore, by doing Pranayam and retaining air in the lungs for a longer time, we reduce the total number of breaths during the day. This will help us to increase longevity.

There are three types of pranayama breathing. We already said them in the introduction, now we develop them. Try these types of breathing to feel them in yourself:

Sit in a meditation pose with crossed legs and hands resting on legs in the meditation pose.

- **Abdominal breathing**

Abdominal breathing is the most common; it is the one we do unconsciously.

When you breathe in, the lower part of the lungs that fill with air moves the diaphragm down, and you can see how the abdomen swells. Pranayama consists of controlling the breath so that the air that fills the lungs is introduced slowly.

Keep your abdominal muscles relaxed, inhaling and expelling the air through your nose. You can place a hand on your belly to feel the movements.

- **Chest breathing**

When taking such a breath, you will notice movement in the ribs as the rib cage expands. To notice this type of breathing to the maximum, force your abs and breathe. By putting tension on the abdominals, you prevent the belly from expanding, and thus the part that swells is the thorax.

- **Clavicular breathing**

It is produced by filling the upper part of the lungs with air. Maybe you have never heard of this type of breathing, so pay close attention, that also the movement in the clavicles is very subtle.

86

Lift your collarbones as you take in air, but do not move your shoulders. Have you tried it? I already told you it was subtle. It is also not very common. It is only mentioned because it does matter if it accompanies the other two types of breathing.

A Set of Pranayama Exercises

Now I am going to explain my set of Pranayam yoga. You can start with Surya Namaskar and any other mentioned asanas to warm up and get rid of extra energy. It can be undoubtedly okay if you just want to do Pranayam yoga.

1.Deep breathing exercise I:

- Sit in a meditation pose and deep breath through your nose with the expansion of your chest.
- Slowly breath out through your nose with your mouth closed.
- Only use the nose for this breathing exercise.
- Repeat 3-5 times (or until you feel settled or calm)

2. Deep breathing exercise II:

- Sit in meditation pose, and deep breath in through your nose
- curl your lips like a whistle
- breathe out slowly through your mouth.
- Repeat 3-5 times.

3. Ujjayi:

This Pranayama exercise is to activate thyroid glands:

- sit on your yoga mat in a meditation pose.
- Breathe in with the glottis (upper part of the throat) with a humming sound while keeping your mouth closed.
- Hold your breath and lower your head to touch your chin to your chest.
- Hold the air as long as you can.

- Lift your head up and close your right nostril withy o u r finger, and exhale the air through the left.

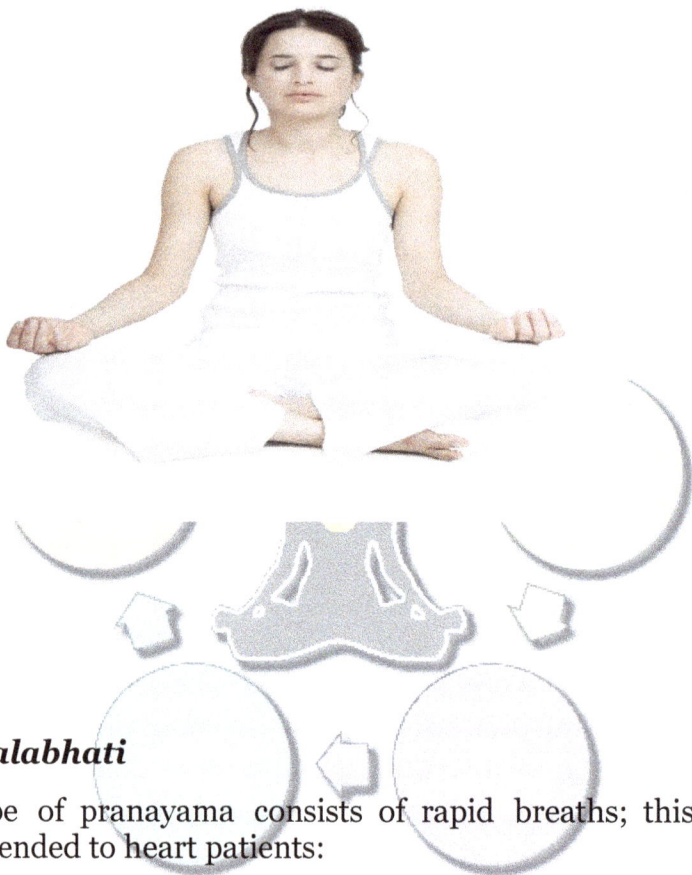

4. *Kapalabhati*

This type of pranayama consists of rapid breaths; this is not recommended to heart patients:

- This is breathing in and out with your abdomen
- Expel the air sharply. It is achieved by the abdominals' rapid contraction, which causes the violent expulsion of air, and by projecting the air into the nostrils (as when blowing).
- In this, you are only focusing on exhalation with force; inhalation is automatic happen.
- Approximately 50 cycles per minute are performed. (check online videos if not sure)

5. Solar Breathing

Close your left nostril, inhale through the right nostril and exhale through it whilst counting 1 to 4.

The right nostril is connected with the sun (known as Pingala Nadi in Yoga) inhaling and exhaling will produce heat in the body. This pranayama is beneficial in cold countries or in winter and monsoon seasons.

6. Lunar Breathing

- Close your right nostril and now inhale and exhale through the left nostril whilst counting as above.
- The left nostril relates to the moon (known as Ida in yoga), producing coolness in the body. Thus, useful in high fever, sunstroke, and the summer season.

7. Anulom Vilom (balancing the heat and cold)

This exercise has magical power and unlimited benefits. This exercise only connects directly to the brain; it relaxes the brain for a few minutes. Anulom-Vilom is a combination of Lunar and solar breathing. That means it regulates the body temperature and keeps us healthy in all seasons. This exercise is done like this:

- Close your right nostril, inhale through the left nostril. Hold the air. Close your left and exhale to the right.
- Now close the left nostril, inhale from the right. Hold the air. Close your right nostril and exhale to the left.
- Keep your eyes closed and focus on your brain; maintain your rhythm for 10-15 minutes.
- While focusing on your brain, imagine that positive energy is going into your brain and deleting all negative, sad, corrupt, unwanted and junk files of your brain.
- The most significant benefit of this exercise is that you cannot think anything else when maintaining the rhythm(cycle).

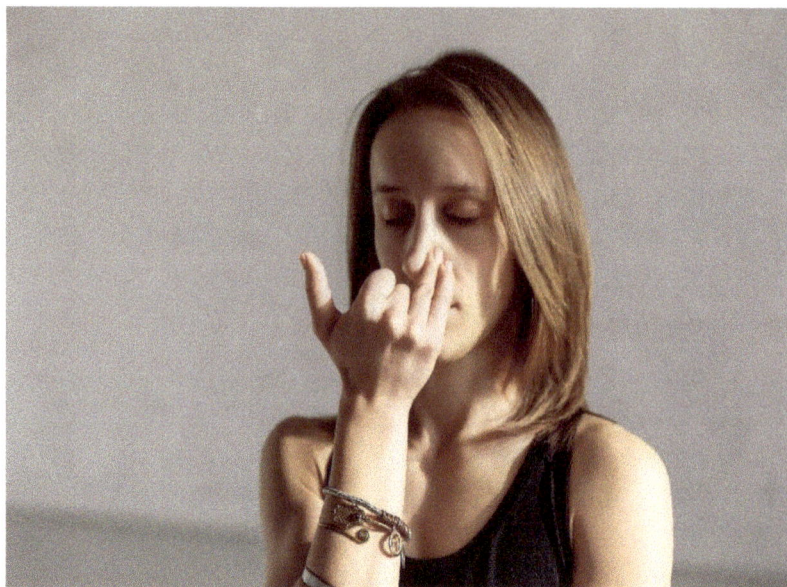

The best thing about this pranayama is that you can do it anytime and anywhere while waiting in the car to collect someone, listening to the radio, and lying on the bed.

You can do this pranayama before going to a meeting; it can improve your creativity and enhance your quick-thinking power. If you are nervous before the interview, try to do this pranayama; you will feel refreshed and energetic. If you are suffering from insomnia, do this while lying on the bed. I am giving my 20 years of testimony for it.

As you might know, our brain is basically symmetrical, spilt into the middle to the right and left hemisphere. The left side of the brain controls the movement of the right side of the body, and the right side of the brain controls the movement of the left side of the body. By this pranayama yoga, we give oxygen to both sides of the brain and indirectly to the whole body.

The other benefits of this pranayama yoga are –

> ➤ It promotes overall wellbeing.
> ➤ It improves our ability to focus and concentrate.
> ➤ It improves fine-motor and gross-motor coordination.
> ➤ It increases respiratory strength and endurance.
> ➤ It restores balance in the left and right hemispheres of the brain.
> ➤ It rejuvenates the nervous system and removes toxins from the brain.
> ➤ It reduces stress, anxiety, frustration and depression.
> ➤ It helps in controlling high blood pressure.
> ➤ It increases positivity and helps to get rid of negative thoughts.
> ➤ It refreshes, reboots and restarts the brain for new learning.
> ➤ It relaxes our brain within a few minutes.
> ➤ It helps to stay away from seasonal diseases and illnesses.

8.Bhramari (buzzing bee)

While sitting in a meditation pose, keep your back and neck straight. Place your thumbs in your ears (pressing the ear tubercle's middle outer part against the ear opening to completely block the ears), three fingers on the eyes and one finger on the forehead.

Breath-in and then breath-out with buzzing Om sound. Remember to keep your mouth closed. Then, try to repeat five times. In Bhramari, the vibration sound produced is very soothing, so this practice eases mental tension and anxiety and helps reduce irritability.

9.Om chanting (Meditation exercise)

Sit in a meditation pose with your back and neck straight, your hands are resting on your legs, and your thumb is touching your index finger. Inhale and then exhale with Om sound. O – should be 30 % and mmm - 70% to create a positing and vibrating sound in the body.

10. Shavasana- (corpse pose)

It is ideal to finish exercises or Yoga with Shavasana to regain energy.

Lie down in a comfortable position, legs wide open and hands wide open at the side in a comfortable position. Count 5 to 1, on one close, your eyes; bring your focus straight down towards your feet and relax it. Then, slowly moving your focus upwards (feet-ankles, shins, calves, knees, thighs, hips – relax your lower back, upper back –relax your abdomen, chest, shoulders- relax your elbows, wrists, fingers, and thumbs – relax your skull, neck, face, and eyes and finally your head and your brain), relax your whole body and take 10 deep breath in and out. Try to beath in from the top of the head and breath out through your toes.

This will relax your whole body and fill you with energy.

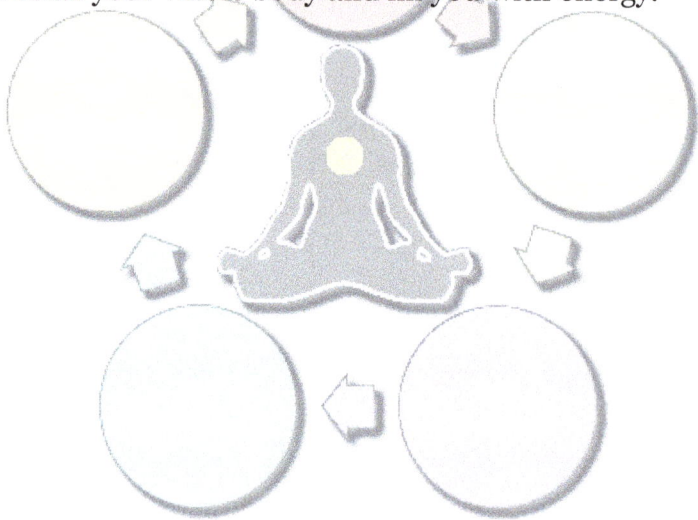

CONCLUSION

When it comes to yoga, the practises have changed over time, but these are ancient practices. Yoga in modern times now focuses on relaxation and focus techniques to stimulate physical energy and spiritual peace.

Ancient yoga dealt less with fitness and more with mental focus and spiritual energy expansion. Then, 2000 years ago, the Yoga Sutra, now considered the ultimate yoga practice guide, came into practice.

Depending on what people want from it and the current fitness level, there are many different yoga types. However, some individuals choose to substitute conventional treatment for yoga conditions, preventing the necessary care from being given to a person.

People with certain conditions should approach yoga slowly and with caution. Although Pranayama Yoga suits everyone. It can be introduced as a beginner to advance level. Breathing is our birthright, and breathing deep is our purpose of life.

A balanced and active lifestyle can be helped by yoga.

References

Health in your hand by Devendra Vora

Center for Mindfulness (CFM). (2005). Mindfulness-based stress reduction program. Retrieved on November 30, 2005, from www.mbsr.org.

Chaline, E. (2001). The simple path to yoga. London: MQ Publications Limited.

Travis, F., Arenander, A., & DuBois, D. (2004). Psychological and physiological characteristics of a proposed object-referral/self-referral continuum of self-awareness. Consciousness and Cognition, 13, 401- 420.

Khan A, Leventhal RM, Khan SR, Brown WA. The severity of depression and response to antidepressants and placebo: an analysis of the Food and Drug Administration database. J Clin Psychopharmacol.2002

Nagarathna R, Nagendra HR. Yoga for anxiety and depression. Bangalore: Swami Vivekananda Yoga Prakashana; 2001.

Woodyard C. Exploring the therapeutic effects of yoga and its ability to increase the quality of life. International Journal of Yoga. 2011

Sengupta P. Health impacts of yoga and pranayama: a state-of-the-art review. Int J Prev Med. 2011;3(7):444–458.

Banerjee B, Vadiraj HS, Ram A, et al. Effects of an integrated yoga program modulating psychological stress and radiation-induced genotoxic stress in breast cancer patients undergoing radiotherapy. Integr Cancer Ther. 2007;6(3):242–250.

Kappmeier K. L., and D. M. Ambrosini. Instructing Hatha Yoga. Champaign, IL: Human Kinetics; 2006

Budilovsky, J., E. Adamson, and C. Flynn. The Complete Idiot's Guide to Yoga. 4th ed. New York, NY: Penguin Group; 2006

Kaminoff, L., and A. Matthews. Yoga Anatomy. 2nd ed. Champaign, IL: Human Kinetics; 2012

International Journal of Yoga

Your Yoga Schedule

Day	Time	Yoga Poses	✔ ☺

Day	Time	Yoga Poses	✅ / ☺

Day	Time	Yoga Poses	✅ ☺

Day	Time	Yoga Poses	✔ 😊

If you like our book, please rate our effort by giving a review on Amazon.

OR

Visit our website for further publications

www.newbeepublication.com

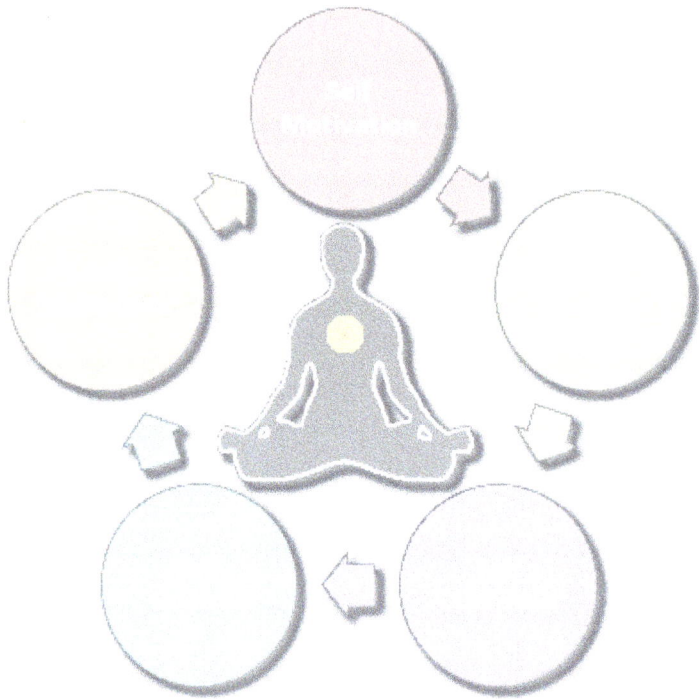

www.ingramcontent.com/pod-product-compliance
Lightning Source LLC
Chambersburg PA
CBHW041929260326
41914CB00009B/1238